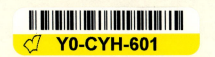

Transnational Aging and Reconfigurations of Kin Work

Global Perspectives on Aging

Sarah Lamb, *Series Editor*

This series publishes books that will deepen and expand our understanding of age, aging, and late life in the United States and beyond. The series focuses on anthropology while being open to ethnographically vivid and theoretically rich scholarship in related fields, including sociology, religion, cultural studies, social medicine, medical humanities, gender and sexuality studies, human development, and cultural gerontology. Books will be aimed at students, scholars, and occasionally the general public.

Jason Danely, *Aging and Loss: Mourning and Maturity in Contemporary Japan*
Parin Dossa and Cati Coe, eds., *Transnational Aging and Reconfigurations of Kin Work*

Transnational Aging and Reconfigurations of Kin Work

EDITED BY PARIN DOSSA AND CATI COE

RUTGERS UNIVERSITY PRESS

NEW BRUNSWICK, CAMDEN, AND NEWARK, NEW JERSEY, AND LONDON

Library of Congress Cataloging-in-Publication Data
Names: Dossa, Parin Aziz, 1945– editor. | Coe, Cati, editor.
Title: Transnational aging and reconfigurations of kin work /
edited by Parin Dossa and Cati Coe.
Description: New Brunswick, New Jersey : Rutgers University Press, 2017. | Series: Global
perspectives on aging | Includes bibliographical references and index.
Identifiers: LCCN 2016024607 | ISBN 9780813588087 (hardback) | ISBN 9780813588070
(pbk.) | ISBN 9780813588094 (e-book (epub))
Subjects: LCSH: Older people—Employment. | Age and employment. | Intergenerational
relations. | Older immigrants. | Kinship. | BISAC: SOCIAL SCIENCE / Emigration &
Immigration. | FAMILY & RELATIONSHIPS / Aging. | POLITICAL SCIENCE /
Globalization. | SOCIAL SCIENCE / Anthropology / Cultural.
Classification: LCC HD6280 .T73 2017 | DDC 331.3/98—dc23
LC record available at https://lccn.loc.gov/2016024607

A British Cataloging-in-Publication record for this
book is available from the British Library.

∞ The paper used in this publication meets the requirements
of the American National Standard for Information Sciences—
Permanence of Paper for Printed Library Materials, ANSI Z39.48-1992.

www.rutgersuniversitypress.org

Manufactured in the United States of America

To
Grandmothers
Mothers and Aunts
All Our Kin

CONTENTS

PART THREE
Aging, Kin Work, and Migrant Trajectories

Transnational Aging and Reconfigurations of Kin Work

Introduction

Transnational Aging and Reconfigurations of Kin Work

PARIN DOSSA AND CATI COE

The living room of Parin Dossa is embellished with several pieces of embroidery given to her by study participants. One wall hanging stands out. It is from Noor, a sixty-six-year-old woman who lives with her married son and his three children in metropolitan Vancouver. Comprising a motif of flowers and abstract designs in varied shades of color, it is a product of Noor's varied experiences—through village life, the market economy, the Iranian Revolution, and migration—which she recounted as follows:

> I was born in the village of Masouleh [in Iran]. I only studied until grade six. There were no schools after this grade in my village. My father said, "You must have some useful skill." He asked my aunt to teach me how to do embroidery. I learned different patterns for cushion coverings, tablecloths, dresses, wall hangings, and so many other things. When I got married at the age of sixteen, I moved to Shiraz. My husband had a large family. My in-laws liked that I was good at embroidery work. When the prices started going up, my in-laws made me do embroidery work for sale. I was not happy as I had to work for ten hours a day. My eyes would water. Only when factory-made embroidery became popular could I slow down. Machine-stitched embroidered work is cheaper. After the Revolution we had to move to Canada. My son worked for the Shah. It was not safe for us to stay there. Over the years, I had collected all kinds of embroidered pieces. I could bring some. I left other pieces with my sister in Iran. I have told her to give these out to our families who now live in the United States and in Australia. I have kept a few pieces for my grandchildren. This way my family can remember me.

Noor's father could not have imagined that the skill that he encouraged his daughter to acquire from her aunt would be used in her old age in a faraway place. Noor's narrative indicates that the fine pieces of embroidered work in Iranian homes in Canada did not merely constitute part of the décor. They are a way older women have sustained their families over the years. They illustrate that older women have moved across geographic spaces. Noor's embroidered work is not frozen in time and space; rather, it is activated in the present transnationally, across and between nation-states. It has circulated within her homeland and its people's diaspora, providing connection among family members dispersed geographically and across generations. Using her embroidery threads, Noor stitches together strands of her lived life.

The goal of this volume is to document the social and emotional contributions of older persons in settings shaped by migration: in their everyday lives, in domestic and community spaces, and in the context of intergenerational relationships and diasporas. As with Noor's embroidery, much of the work of older men and women in transnational families is oriented toward supporting, connecting, and maintaining kin members and kin relationships, which we consider to be kin work, the work that enables a family to reproduce and regenerate itself across the generations. This volume examines the variety of kin work done by older men and women as transnational migrants to sustain their families emotionally and materially over time: from childcare to paid labor. Kin work also includes more subtle forms of care such as memorializing efforts.

Examining the kin work of older adults in transnational families provides one analytic window on how families are managing the exclusions and expulsions of globalization. Kin members, labor markets, and states—the latter particularly in their immigration policies, pension and social security regimes, and childcare support—all affect the kin work that older men and women assume and enact. Furthermore, the kin work of the aged has implications for their own aging trajectories, identities and status, networks of relationships, and migration and mobility. Social and economic inequality is visible in the intimacies of family life and the efforts of families to survive and sustain themselves.

The Significance of Aging to Studies of Transnational Migration

Most current work on transnationalism—the connections and identifications maintained across borders—has overlooked the significance of older men and women (for important exceptions, see Baldassar and Merla 2013; Cole and Durham 2007; Lamb 2009). Studies of transnationalism have emphasized its importance in fostering social and cultural ties (Georges 1990), generating economic activity (Portes 2003) and activating social and political movements in homelands and their diasporas (Fouron and Schiller 2002; Rouse 1992). However, despite their insights, the literature on transnational migration has under-played the transformative work of older adults and the ways that they and those they care for are affected by growing global inequality and precarity.

Common assumptions hold that those involved in transnational migra-tion are only those who cross borders and that those who cross borders are young and able bodied. The social invisibility of older men and women is rep-licated in immigration policies that do not acknowledge their contributions to familial, cultural, and economic reproduction. Such social invisibility has real consequences, as border crossing is not free flowing but politically deter-mined. Countries that enjoy global hegemony such as the United States, Great Britain, Canada, Western Europe, and Australia have tightly controlled borders with specific criteria for who can enter based on a person's possession of skill, capital, or family connection (Andall 2013; Balgamwalla 2014; Boucher 2007). These criteria often exclude older persons; they are not perceived to be workers, but rather, the dependents of wage earners and a drain on national resources as users of social and health services. For example, older men and women in Australia, Canada, and in the European Union are allocated to the immigra-tion category of being sponsored by adult migrant children. As the chapters by Neda Deneva, Yanqiu Rachel Zhou, and Mushira Moshin Khan and Karen Koya-bashi (this volume) illustrate, the immigration category of sponsorship renders aging persons legally and socially dependent on their adult children, resulting in a reconfiguration of kin relationships, roles in households, and aging tra-jectories. Furthermore, by excluding nonworking members of migrant families, and separating family members across borders (Coe 2013; Hahamovitch 2011), countries receiving immigrants can outsource some of the costs of these fami-lies' educational and health services to their countries of origin. In migrants' home countries, aging persons may be central to the care of those left behind, including the children of migrants (Deneva, this volume; Yarris, this volume). The critical work of older people in regenerating families socially, emotionally, and economically through family narratives, religious instruction, memory work, wage labor, cooking, and childcare remains overlooked and unrecognized by states.

Some older men and women were migrants in their youth and have grown old in the country of migration. Some aged migrants retire to their home coun-tries or where their children are located. Others accompany or follow their migrant relatives in middle or old age, through family sponsorship or other means. Still others remain in the country of origin. As Georges Fouron and Nina Glick Schiller (2002) have noted, both those who go and those who stay are involved in and affected by transnational migration. For those who stay in the home country, the global discourse on the so-called crisis of aging defines them as a burden on society and family, missing their absent children and reliant on remittances. Instead, ethnographic research has shown that those who remain behind may be involved in reverse social and financial remittances (Mazzucato 2008b), such as caring for their grandchildren, the children of migrants (Bastia 2009; Rae-Espinoza 2011; Yarris, this volume); supporting their migrant children financially (Baldassar, this volume); or giving religious or social donations in migrants' names to enable migrants to maintain a social presence in the hometown (Small 1997). These highly active roles of supporting migrants and sustaining their connections to their hometowns are not usually recognized by the extensive scholarship on remittances, which views those who remain behind as dependent on wage-earning migrants. In this volume, we delineate the multiple ways in which older adults contribute to family reproduction in contexts where labor markets and states are not sufficient to meet family needs.

How do we validate the life experiences of people dismissed as socially and economically irrelevant? In her work *Feminism and Anthropology* (1988), Henrietta Moore addresses this question in relation to women. She traces the ambiguity of the place of women in social anthropology to the descriptive presence of women in ethnographic accounts, on the one hand, and their absence at the level of theory and analysis, on the other. She notes that the mere addition of "women to traditional anthropology would not resolve the problem of women's analytical 'invisibility'" (1988, 3). As with gender, aging members of transnational families cannot merely be added empirically to the burgeoning literature on transnationalism. Rather, how difference is generated through the category of age and how aging may be distinct processes for differently positioned persons need to be brought to the fore of transnationalism. In addition to complicating our understanding of transnationalism, we find that a focus on transnational aging generates new thinking about the past, the life course, intergenerational effects, cohorts, and the habitus.

Barbara Myerhoff's ethnography *Number Our Days* (1978) is inspirational in showing how migration and aging are reconceptualized when considered together. Contrary to her expectations, Myerhoff found a vibrant community among the Holocaust survivors who participated in a Jewish senior center in California. She notes, "Center people, like so many of the elderly, were very fond of reminiscing and storytelling, eager to be heard from, eager to relate parts of their life history. More afraid of oblivion than pain or death, they always sought opportunities to become visible" (1978, 33). Their anxiety for visibility and attention at the end of life was in some sense a response to their social isolation, including their adult children's neglect of them in a new land, where their wisdom and Yiddish language fluency did not seem relevant. Being old in a beach community in California, where youth is celebrated, is different than being old in a shtetl in Eastern Europe (Myerhoff and Littman 1977). The significance Judaism places on memory helped sustain these older Jews' personal projects of being remembered by their friends and family and made the past come alive in the present.[1] Although the term "transnationalism" was not in currency at the time, Myerhoff's work (1978) highlighted three questions relevant to current studies of transnational migration and aging: (a) What is it like to leave one's place of birth and grow old in a new land? (b) How do rituals and celebrations keep alive historical memories for younger generations diverted by what is new? (c) How does the meaning of old age and elderhood vary in different social and geographical locations?

Like Myerhoff's ethnography, the chapters in this volume analyze the effect of temporalities on migration and migrants. Many of the chapters consider the ways that past events, including histories of migration in the life course of migrants and nonmigrants, affect contemporary experiences of mobility. The chapters by Delores V. Mullings and Cati Coe examine the ways that immigrants' employment pathways into low-paid, low-skilled work affect them in old age, raising questions of incorporation in and exclusion from their countries of migration. More subtly, with a concern for intergenerational effects, Kristin Elizabeth Yarris examines the ways that grandmothers caring for their grandchildren, the children of migrants, interpret their previous experiences of the migration of a loved one—including their husband and children. This interpretation frames how the caregivers in the home country anticipate the impending migration of the grandchild they care for, when he or she joins the migrant parent abroad. Yarris's chapter illustrates intergenerational effects—not only the ways that the old affect the young, but also the ways that the young affect the old. A focus on aging allows us to consider the multiple and complex ways in which the past, present, and future shape each other and how the generations exert influence on each other, in shaping migration decisions, experiences, and trajectories.

Furthermore, a focus on aging draws attention to the ways that the timing and transitions of diverse life courses affect one another, influencing a person's mobility or immobility. As the chapters by Deneva and Zhou explore, aging parents and grandparents travel or stay put in relation not only to their own employment and marital transitions but also to the aging and illness experiences of their own parents, the births and education of grandchildren, and the employment of migrant children. Although all the chapters have some sense of the past, Loretta Baldassar explores this aspect of migration most deeply, with her examination of the care practices of different migrant cohorts across the hundred years of Italian migration to Australia. The exploration of aging makes time, timing, the life course, cohorts, and generations central to transnational migration, when considering how these issues shape migration decisions, cultures of migrations, and the social and emotional effects of transnational migration.

As the chapters in the volume show, studies of aging can raise new questions and offer fresh insights into what it is like to live in a transnational world, regardless of whether older men and women themselves migrate. We argue that merely adding age to the existing youth-centered paradigm of transnational migration will not do justice to the nuanced transnational life worlds of young and old alike. The issue is not merely learning about the age-related predicaments, contradictions, and ambiguities that invariably inform trajectories of migration and nonmigration. Our goal is to acknowledge and examine age—along with time, timing, the life course, and generations—as social forces shaping such predicaments and ambiguities.

The Significance of Transnationalism to Studies of Aging

Just as our understanding of transnational migration is expanded by considering aging and older adults, so too does transnational migration shift our understanding of aging. In this discussion, we draw on earlier theorists of aging, whose work shaped anthropological thinking and focused attention, through their ethnographically rich work, on topics that broadened the discussion of aging beyond a focus on crisis and decline. We have mined these seminal works for their insights at the same time as we point out the ways in which these theories need to be revised and modified in the context of transnational migration. In particular, we think the kin work of older adults gains particular practical and theoretical salience in social contexts where social and familial regeneration is threatened in multiple ways.

In an earlier work, Andrei Simic (1978) offers analytical insights about how the conceptualization of age can vary in different contexts. In non-Western societies, old age is seamlessly integrated into the dynamic evolution of families and communities. Using the metaphor of "aging as a career," Barbara Myerhoff and Andrei Simic note, "Aging cannot be understood in isolation, but rather must be conceived as a product" of the entire lifespan to that point, which has been building over time (1977, 240). Thus, old age is not a separate stage, but rather enfolds childhood, youth, and middle age as part of the life course. In Western contexts, however, older adults, like children, may be secluded in age-specific institutions and contexts, such as nursing homes and retirement communities (Diamond 1992; Gubrium 1975). Thus, the meaning of aging may vary in different social contexts and change with migration.

In *Age and Anthropological Theory*, David Kertzer and Jennie Keith (1984) make similar points. First, they argue that aging must be considered in dynamic terms. In other words, there is no particular age range when people are categorized as old. For example, in Ghana, it is people's bodily weakness or strength that are considered significant for their aging, rather than the number of years they have been alive (van der Geest 2002). In some communities, generation and birth order may be more significant than absolute age (Fortes 1984). Furthermore, aging and the status of elderhood do not always go hand in hand. Maurice Bloch notes that in Madagascar, "Men slip into the role of being an elder more easily and more clearly than women, although women may also attain the status of elder, only more rarely and more uncertainly" (1998, 183). Elderhood itself is dynamic and performed: men adopt particular ways of speaking, using formalized language highly decorated with proverbs and quotations when they perform the role of a respected elder; in more private contexts, they do not always speak in this way.

Aging is a continuum and culturally it may even extend beyond our physical lives into the realm of ancestors and memory. Among the Beng of Côte d'Ivoire, as in other parts of West Africa, the spirits of ancestors may return in the bodies of newborns, and thus babies are constructed as "old" and from the spirit world (Gottlieb 2004). Retirement from purposeful, remunerated activity, rather than age per se, was one sign of old age among aging Puerto Ricans in Harlem, many of whom began working in adolescence (Freidenberg 2000). Governments emphasize the significance of age in measuring identity and status through birth registration, identification documents, forms that require one's birth date or age, and census records (Ariès 1962). They also mediate the definition of old age through their social welfare projects: for example, in the United States, the age at which one becomes eligible for Social Security and Medicare, the government-sponsored pension and health insurance program for older adults, has become the marker of old age (Coe, this volume; Freidenberg 2000; Gilbertson 2009). Like disability and mental illness (Biehl 2005; Livingston 2005), transitions into old age are often mediated by a person's social networks, which enable activity or dependency, good or poor nutrition, and access to medical attention. Thus, it is important to keep in mind that aging is a dynamic process, affected by social contexts.

Secondly, Kertzer and Keith (1978) argue that aging rituals, practices, and social roles are diverse. Aging is significant in a person's life course because age is a principle of social organization. Older persons are not simply defined by their aging bodies, but also by the representations of old age and aged people (Cohen 1998). For example, in the United States, through the discourse on successful aging, older men and women are encouraged to be as vibrant and independent as possible through their individual efforts (Lamb 2014). In Botswana, in contrast, receiving care from others is a sign of being respected and having lived a life of helping others (Livingston 2005). For the Dutch, living independently means living apart from adult children; whereas among Italians, it means relying on family and not the state (Baldassar, Wilding, and Baldock 2007). Among the Fulbe in northern Cameroon (Regis 2003), women's aging allows them to become more pious and to garner the respect associated with Muslim religious practice, a respect denied them when they were giving birth and raising children. Older men and women are expected to act their age. Because aging processes are diverse in different sociocultural contexts, some aging transnational migrants may nostalgically contrast old age in the homeland as a time of ease, respect, and social connection with the difficulties and loneliness of growing old in the country of migration (Coe, this volume; Gardner 2002).

Finally, in our delineation of the human life course, we need to bear in mind that biological aging is affected by sociality, financial resources, and other social factors, as well as being marked differently in different social contexts. "Loneliness kills," many Ghanaians told Cati Coe in explaining why they organized social events for the aged. On the other hand, medicalized situations tend to focus on biological aging in isolation, for the purpose of control and management (Lock 1995). Even contexts that are considered more holistic than hospitals in attending to social relations and ethical values—such as hospice and palliative care—tend to focus on the medical needs of the aging body (Dossa, this volume).

Because age is a principle of social organization, it is deeply rooted in the political economy and can provide a lens through which we can understand social change in today's world. Jennifer Cole and Deborah Durham argue that age mediates "relationships in the family and household, social cohorts across space, and history and change. In the course of these mediations, age links world-historical economic and social change with the intimate spaces of caring and obligation within the family" (2007, 2). Sarah Lamb observes similarly, "Beliefs and practices surrounding aging illuminate much broader sociocultural phenomena, including global cultural and economic flows; the relationships between persons, families and states; the nature of gender; and compelling moral visions of how best to live" (2009, x). Older persons themselves can be agents of social change, she emphasizes. In her ethnographic work carried out in India and the United States, Lamb makes a case for understanding how people translate processes of modernization and globalization into their everyday lives. After all, they themselves are encountering aging and frailty as a new experience personally (Cole 2013). As they age, they create new meanings of what it means to be old, perhaps making their vulnerability into a resource (Raffety, this volume).

Because political, social, and economic processes shape family life and intimate relations, looking at the roles, relationships, and activities of older people tells us a great deal about globalization and how it is affecting familial and social reproduction (Cole and Durham 2007). Eleonore Kofman notes, "The extent to which one is able to physically and socially reproduce families and households depends in turn on rights of mobility, immigration, residence and citizenship status" (2012, 154). Deborah Boehm (2012), likewise, in her beautiful and nuanced ethnography of Mexican transnational families, shows how state policies affect who can move and who remains behind and thus affect intimate relations between parents and children and between spouses. In this volume, we argue that the effortful and engaged activity of older persons in transnational families is a key site for understanding how capitalist labor markets and neoliberal state policies impact family life. The labor of older people in transnational families renders visible the workings of structural forces whose power, in a transnational context, cannot be underestimated. Through the concept of kin work, we turn now to delineating the contours and implications of this labor for selfhood, relationships, and social identity.

Kin Work and Transnational Aging

We find the concept of kin work, as defined and elaborated by Carol Stack and Linda M. Burton (1993), remains valuable in describing and analyzing the labor of older men and women in transnational families. By their definition, kin work is "the labor and tasks that a family needs to accomplish to survive from generation to generation" (157). According to Stack and Burton,

> kin-work regenerates families, maintains lifetime continuities, sustains intergenerational responsibilities, and reinforces shared values. It encompasses, for example, all of the following: family labor for reproduction; intergenerational care for children and dependents; economic survival including wage and nonwage labor; family migration and migratory labor designated to send home remittances; and strategic support for networks of kin extending across regions, state lines, and nations. (160–161)

There are several useful features of their definition that we wish to emphasize. First, it puts unpaid work—such as childcare, elder care, and domestic chores—on an equal footing with paid work that brings cash income into the family; both kinds of labor are ways that families maintain themselves over time (Safri and Graham 2010). Western feminism has long highlighted the value of unpaid care work and household labor—often done by women and performed in the private domain—as critical for the reproduction of households (for a recent overview, see Weeks 2011); as a result, some scholars call it reproductive labor (Meillassoux 1972; Glenn 1992). The invisibility and unpaid character of reproductive labor are often contrasted with the visibility and valuation of productive labor, compensated by a cash wage and associated with the public, male domain. Stack and Burton's formulation, in which both productive and reproductive labor support kin, allows us to distance ourselves from dichotomies of private/public, paid/unpaid, valued/not-valued, and male/female to examine how people are involved in sustaining their families and the cultural valuations of their labor within their particular social milieu.

Secondly, Stack and Burton emphasize that kin work is not tied to households or shared residence, but can happen "across regions, state lines, and nations" (1993, 161). Migration is an important feature of economic survival for families today. Such migration can be across international borders or different regions within the same country. Many families today find that to sustain themselves, some or all members have to travel to live elsewhere. Many studies of transnational families show how kin work and households are distributed across geographically dispersed locations (Boehm 2012; Coe 2013; Olwig 2007). For example, children of migrants, rather than accompanying a parent or both parents abroad, may remain behind in their grandparents' care, with the household supported by the migrant's remittances (Parreñas 2004; Yarris 2014b). Such arrangements may result in reconfigurations of kin roles and relationships; for example, grandmothers may be called "mothers" by their grandchildren with whom they reside, as an attempt to normalize a situation that outsiders see as problematic (Rae-Espinoza 2011). Or migrant mothers may try to redefine what being a "good mother" means, emphasizing that mothering means financially supporting their children, rather than being present on a daily basis to sing the child to sleep or nurse the wounds from minor accidents (Parreñas 2004; Schmalzbauer 2004). Elder care by migrants may become more about personal connection and maintenance of a relationship across distance, rather than helping with daily activities or household chores, which may be delegated to proxy caregivers (Baldassar, this volume). In this volume as a whole, we are interested in how families use their mobility to sustain themselves and others, and how such mobility reconfigures the labor that maintains families.

We can see how Noor's embroidery constitutes kin work in several ways. First, when she was a young woman in Iran, it allowed her to make a living. As a result, it made her more attractive to her in-laws, with whom she lived, helping to solidify her marriage. Second, after her migration, her finished embroidery functioned as a valued gift that knit together family members dispersed across Iran, Canada, and Australia, keeping alive their sense of connection and mutual feeling, which Marshall Sahlins (2010, 2011) sees as central to kinship. Her embroidery also makes the homeland visible both for those who were born and grew up there and for those who have never seen it, on the walls within which each family member carries out the activities of daily life. Thus, her embroidery re-creates a sense of home—a home that is dispersed. It helps generate a transnational home for a transnational family. The literary writer Salman Rushdie observed, "The past is a country from which we have all immigrated, that its loss is part of our common humanity" and "this part of our heritage can only be recovered through the meaning we build through scraps, memories, and everyday realities" (1991, 12). It is through "scraps, memories, and everyday realities" that many aged migrants maintain generational legacies and relationships that recuperate the past and socially regenerate the present (Cole and Durham 2007). Kin work includes memorializing projects and re-creations of home and the homeland through music and food (Dossa, this volume); photographs that recall kin dispersed across the globe and connect new generations to place and people who are gone (Dossa, this volume); and narratives of migration that seek to maintain relationships between migrant parents and their children who remain behind (Yarris, this volume). Although kin of whatever generation and age can help keep family memories alive and regenerate social relations in the present, older men and women in transnational families seem especially sought out and engaged in this kind of kin work as a result of their social roles and experiences.

Two other concepts accompany Stack and Burton's understanding of kin work: kin time and kin-scription. Kin time is the sequencing and timing of the tasks and labor required to sustain a family over time. The timing of kin work may not always be synchronized across multiple life courses, and may be the source of tensions and conflicts that reconfigure the social identities of kin members. Take the example of Fatme cited by Deneva (2012), who left her home and factory work in Bulgaria to take care of her nine-year-old grandson in Spain so that her daughter could take up work in a restaurant. Shortly thereafter, her son, who had moved to Portugal, pressured her to take care of his teenage children; sons have greater claims than daughters to their mother's reproductive labor and greater obligations to provide support in the future. Wanting to meet her care obligations to her son, Fatme went to Portugal only to find that the teenagers did not really need supervision and the work her son had arranged for her—picking orchard fruit—was onerous. She returned to her daughter in Spain a week later, only to find out that her daughter in Spain had lost her job while Fatme was away and no longer needed help with childcare. Fatme returned to her hometown to work in a sewing workshop, having been labeled "a problem grandmother" by her relatives. Fatme's performance of her social identity as an elder worthy of respect is bound up with her kin work, which is dependent on the timing of transitions in the life courses of her children, including their own employment and fertility trajectories. Similarly, Coe (2016) argues that care requires a synchronization or social entrainment of temporalities across multiple life courses. A Ghanaian female migrant in the United States found it difficult to coordinate her life course with those of her dying mother and her adolescent nephews who were then living with her mother in Ghana. The distance made it hard to monitor and evaluate the course of her mother's illness and decline. Furthermore, American regulations on international adoption made it impossible to bring her adolescent nephews to the United States in the wake of her mother's death. Thus, kin work is dependent on kin timing, or the coordination of the timing of events—whether birth, schooling, employment, illness, or death—across multiple life courses.

Kin-scription is how particular members of the family become conscripted to particular kinds of kin work based on cultural scripts about family roles, which are often based on gender and age. For example, an ethnographic study by Stack (1996) shows how the migrant daughters of frail African American older adults were kin-scripted to return home to the southern United States, while migrant sons were less likely to be called home in midcareer. Numerous chapters in the volume discuss kin-scription by the aged and kin-scription into elder care. The chapters in this first section of this volume, by Deneva, Zhou, and Kristin Elizabeth Yarris, show that older women are often kin-scripted to the work of providing unpaid childcare for their grandchildren, to allow a migrant parent to work. This kin-scription can happen by leaving children behind in the care of their grandparents, or by migrant children sponsoring their parents' migration to join them abroad. In the second section, Erin Raffety discusses the way that older women in China become involved in foster parenting as a way to obtain income, companionship, and status. In the same section, Khan and Kobayashi describe how South Asian daughters and daughters-in-law in Canada manage their kin-scription to elder care, through the idealized roles of the dutiful daughter and obedient wife, despite the increased demands of work and children.

Thus, we build on Stack and Burton's concept of kin work in ways that we think are in line with their thinking. Kin work brings into relief two critical issues for the study of transnational aging. First, it allows us to explore the complex migration trajectories of older women and men in the context of their social relationships and networks, including how their migrations are part of the labor that sustains families. Second, kin work allows us to document the reproductive labor of older migrants as having the same value as waged work. We consider this to be significant because those considered as the elderly are often considered to be a discrete constituency who are recipients of services, rather than contributors of labor (waged or otherwise), as we discuss further in the next section. Making tangible what may otherwise remain elusive, we argue that it is through kin work that older persons can be recognized as a powerful social force.

Kin Work and Reciprocity

Although wage labor and market relations may be one of the factors that help to sustain families over time, material, economic, and social resources are not generally distributed by and between kin through direct, immediate, com- modified exchanges. Instead, kin distribute these resources through alterna- tive, longer-term circuits of valuation based on sharing and cooperation (Folbre 2001, 2008; Sahlins 2004; Zelizer 2005). The sharing of resources is moti- vated by emotion and obligation resulting from previous social and material exchanges. Because resources are shared between people who have a sense of connection to one another (or would like to), Noor's gifts of embroidery do not only distribute valued material resources, which might be sold in the market- place, but also index and maintain kin relationships. Her embroidery maintains a sense of home among widely dispersed kin. Because exchanges between kin operate according to a different logic than capitalism or wage labor (Gibson- Graham 2006; Sahlins 2010, 2011), they can serve as a safety net for individuals who are no longer able to engage in productive labor or are excluded from the exchanges and relations dominated by capitalism (Meillassoux 1972; Stack 1974). Because labor markets sometimes discriminate against older men and women (Neumark and Button 2014), kin exchanges may become more central to their personal wellbeing and they may engage in greater effort to maintain them.[2]

Because aged men and women may no longer be part of the productive workforce, we might expect them to be recipients, rather than givers, in the exchanges between kin. Instead, the chapters in this volume show the need to complicate this image of the aged. First, as the scholarship on gift giving shows (Bourdieu 1977; Mauss 1990), gifts generate obligations for others to reciprocate in the future. In the words of Parker Shipton, they create entrustments: "Entrust- ment implies an obligation, but not necessarily an obligation to repay like with like, as a loan might imply. Whether an entrustment or transfer is returnable in kind or in radically different form—be it economic, political, symbolic, or some mixture of these—is a matter of cultural context and strategy" (2007, 11). Thus, because gifts are socially constructed as entrustments, it is difficult to deter- mine who is the beneficiary or recipient, and who is the benefactor or giver, in kin work. The aged are not simply recipients of care or cash; rather, their kin work in the past may have created an entrustment which others reciprocate in the present. As a Ghanaian proverb states, "Someone cared for you while your teeth were coming in [as a baby]; look after that person when his/her teeth are falling out [in old age]" (Coe 2013, 61).[3] Furthermore, as the chapter by Deneva (this volume) shows, older women from Bulgaria hope to create an entrustment in the future by their labor in the present: by taking care of their grandchildren, thus allowing their adult children to engage in paid labor, they hope their children will care for them when they need help. Changes in care result in changes in other exchanges, such as inheritance: Baldassar (this vol- ume) shows how migrant children in Australia may give up their parental inher- itance to siblings who remain behind in Italy and provided personal care to aging parents. Likewise, although the youngest son in Bulgaria usually inherits the parents' land and house and takes care of his aging parents, the migration of youngest sons means that no one may want to inherit and no one may feel obligated to provide elder care (Deneva, this volume). Entrustments are inherently asymmetrical and uneven, dependent on need and the capacity to give (Baldassar and Merla 2014). Entrustments are also precarious and dependent on ongoing exchanges.

Because entrustments need to be maintained, as ethnographic work on aging shows quite strongly, older men and women make efforts to be givers, as well as recipients, of material and social resources in ongoing exchanges. For example, Emiliana, an older woman profiled in Judith Freidenberg's (2000) study of aging men and women in Spanish Harlem, talks proudly about all the ways she continues to support her relations, despite her economic precarity: she cooks more food than she can eat so she can feed family and friends who drop by unexpectedly; members of the next generation, including her step-children and a nephew, have stayed (illegally) in her subsidized apartment set aside for seniors; and she shares the proceeds of her social security check with others when they are in need. Freidenberg notes, "Emiliana sees herself as a giver regardless of her economic situation, a self-image that has tremendous impact on her dignity and self-respect and makes her central to her personal network" (186). Freidenberg argues that Emiliana engages in these forms of kin work despite her poverty because "giving enhances the predictability of being socially recognized during one's lifetime and compensated in the afterlife" (187). Although we might expect impoverished aged people to be recipients of gifts, they work hard to position themselves as reciprocally engaged with kin and thus socially active. The chapters by Yarris, Raffety, Mullings, and Parin Dossa show older women repositioning themselves as contributors to kin and the nation; through these kin work contributions, they gain a sense of self-worth, social networks, and a place in the world.

Furthermore, older men and women continue to be engaged in forms of productive labor, perhaps part-time, through small-scale entrepreneurial activities, or in the informal economy (Coe, this volume; Deneva, this volume; Freidenberg 2000). The continued involvement in productive labor by relatively healthy older adults, who are sometimes called "the young-old," is partly a way to hedge their bets, should other entrustments fall through, and partly a mode of continued survival. Income from their wage labor may also be disbursed among kin, as an important form of kin work (Deneva, this volume; Mullings, this volume).

Older men and women may receive some income not simply from their current wage labor but also from their previous labor through pensions and social security. Involvement in productive labor in some nation-states allows the aged to receive disbursements pegged to their accumulated wages and years of employment. These payments can seem precarious in an era of neoliberalism and uncertain economic futures. For example, rampant inflation can wipe out the value of pensions, making Russian pensioners dependent on growing their own potatoes for daily meals (Ries 2009). Or, in another example, political officials in the United States have warned that the current social security system will run out of funds in fifteen years, unless changes are made (Foroohar 2014).[4] However, even when a pension or social security income is paltry, in certain contexts it allows aging people to be more financially secure than other impoverished members of their families. Research on old-age pensions in Namibia and South Africa, for example, shows that such payments are disbursed intergenerationally, and across the recipient's kin network (Klocke-Daffa 2014; Lloyd-Sherlock et al. 2012). Thus, like others, the aged may rely on multiple kinds of exchanges with kin, the market, and the state (sometimes multiple states), as a way of coping with personal and familial uncertainty about the future. Yet managing such different kinds of resources may create its own anxiety, as aging men and women wonder where to place their trust, energy, and resources.

In this volume, we focus on the various contributions of older women and men to sustaining transnational families, whether or not they themselves migrate. This approach helps to reverse the perception of older people as mere recipients of familial and state-initiated care, and instead shows the ways that different members of families are kin-scripted into employment and unpaid labor in the collective labor of sustaining families over time. Rejecting the binary of receiving or giving care, we reveal the ways they are intertwined in order to emphasize the active multifaceted labor of older men and women and of their relatives in transnational families. The concept of kin work enhances this emphasis. Our intent is to show how older persons sustain family and community life through "words of wisdom," "scraps" of cloth, anecdotes, prayers, and religious commentary as well as unpaid care work, paid employment, volunteering, and business services, all of which we conceptualize as kin work. The import of this work is realized in light of the fact that the burgeoning literature on transnationalism does not substantively include the experiences and labor of aging and older immigrants.

Case Studies of Transnational Kin Work

The volume illustrates the multiple ways in which members of transnational families are engaged in kin work and care for their members in contexts of expulsion, exclusion, and declining state support for family regeneration in the context of neoliberal capitalism. Older people are recruited into or place themselves into new caregiving roles. Adjustments to intergenerational reciprocity and social status are made, creating new dynamics in families and across the generations. Kin work is shaped by immigration policies; state social support for health, education, and pensions; and the social roles and kin-scripts assigned to and assumed by older adults and others. Case studies explore these issues in both migrant-sending and migrant-receiving countries, and many in both contexts. Migrants are from Bulgaria, China, Ghana, Italy, Jamaica, Nicaragua, South Asia (India and Sri Lanka), the United Kingdom, the United States, and the East African countries of Kenya, Tanzania, and Uganda. They establish lives in Australia, Canada, the Netherlands, Spain, and the United States, and they travel back and forth between their homelands, the countries of migration, and other places where their relatives have settled.

The case studies highlight a range of older adults—from young-old to more frail old to dying, and from impoverished to middle class to wealthy. Some have biological or adopted children and grandchildren; others are childless. Some are married; others have never married or were widowed. We aim to illustrate our general themes across this variety of cases. Some of the chapters focus on older migrants aging in the country of migration where they have lived for a long time; other chapters illustrate elderly migrants who join their migrant children. And in yet other chapters, aging migrants return to their hometown or to a new place entirely. Some aged persons have not moved: they are caring for children who eventually will migrate to join parents or adoptive parents abroad. The chapters mainly concentrate on older women, reflecting the distribution of kin work within families (but see Dossa, this volume; Khan and Kobayashi, this volume).

Part one, "The Kin-scription of Older People into Care," examines the ways that aged persons are scripted into kin work, participating voluntarily in such tasks through kin-scripts and aged roles. The three chapters in this section focus on the recruitment of older women (and their male spouses) by adult children who need help raising their own children, because they are pursuing work and schooling abroad. Deneva explores how older women from Bulgaria are kin-scripted by their migrant sons and daughters to provide childcare, both abroad and in the hometown, as the timing of others' life courses requires. Such kin-scription means the loss of paid employment and state welfare support, and greater dependence on their children as economic providers, which she terms "kinfare." Zhou's chapter explores a similar phenomenon, in which Chinese migrants to Canada ask their parents to join them to provide childcare and other assistance with domestic chores. Such involvement in kin work results in new aging trajectories in which older migrants have to learn "to be an elder in Canada": their senior status matters less in households, they have to do care work and housework, and they are isolated from the wider society. Like

Deneva, Zhou describes how elders adjust to their new roles and documents the new inequalities of familial life.

Yarris also examines grandmothers taking care of their grandchildren, in this case because their daughters have migrated to the United States. However, the primary form of care that she analyzes is not the domestic chores and child-care noted by Deneva and Zhou, but rather the ways that grandmothers try to influence their grandchildren's experiences of mother-child separation through a narrative of family sacrifice, in which all members suffer for a common goal of family well-being. This narrative, which helps maintain children's connection and relationship to their mothers, is constantly under threat by another interpretation of migration, that of abandonment, experienced by the same grandmothers at earlier times of their life, when first their husbands and then their children migrated abroad. Thus, Yarris considers the more affective and emotional side of kin work, in maintaining intergenerational ties, in contrast to the more pragmatic and practical activities performed by grandparents in the chapters by Deneva and Zhou. All three chapters share a similar theme: kinship roles, care, and aged trajectories are being reshaped by the kin-scription of older people into care; these two issues are treated more deeply in parts two and three.

Part two considers how kin relationships and care are being reconfigured in the context of mobility. All three chapters analyze what care means in particular social contexts. In her chapter, Raffety examines how poor older women in China are fostering disabled children, who are later adopted internationally, in the context of changing entrustments between generations that leave the aging adults vulnerable and lonely. Although the older women do not obtain care for themselves through these fosterage relationships, these women enhance their status, social networks, and sense of self-worth by sacrificing for the good of the nation. Despite the ways that older foster mothers are characterized as "backward" and "greedy" by middle-aged care workers at state orphanages and international adoption agencies, Raffety argues that these care workers are facing their own struggles balancing work and childcare and are jealous of the strong emotional bonds between foster mothers and their foster children. As a result, she argues that foster mothers are agents of social change, in creating alternative kinds of kinship, new care norms, and a new basis of status for the aged.

The next two chapters are concerned with how transnational migration changes the kin care *of* the aged, rather than care *by* the aged. Khan and Kobayashi examine how Hindu middle-aged immigrant women from India and Sri Lanka cope with upholding practices of filial obligation in the context of increased work and school burdens in Canada, similar to the middle-aged bureaucrats profiled by Raffety. Living in multigenerational households in Canada, they find themselves having to balance the needs of their children and those of their in-laws and parents. Given the downgrading of their socioeconomic status in Canada, compared to what they experienced in their homelands, they have trouble providing care according to their cultural ideals. The middle-aged women have trouble enumerating the kind of care they provide to aging parents or in-laws in ways intelligible to Canadian statistics, speaking to a more fluid understanding of care.

Baldassar expands on the theme of what care means. Her study examines the different communication technologies used by different migrant cohorts from Italy to Australia, focusing on letters, packages, gifts of photos and other valued items, phone calls, and polymedia through Skype, instant messaging, and chat forums. Just as Yarris expanded notions of care beyond pragmatic, practical chores to migration narratives that shape intergenerational relationships and maintain family closeness, Baldassar considers keeping relationships active to be an important form of care, which migrant children can provide from afar. The polymedia of the contemporary moment allows ambient copresence and care by proxy.

Part three, "Aging, Kin Work, and Migrant Trajectories," focuses on how transnationalism affects aging as a process of the life course. In particular, it examines the ways in which aging is shaped by past life experiences, state policies, and social networks. All these themes have been touched on in other chapters; here, they are examined more systematically and in depth. Coe analyzes the retirement strategies of older Ghanaian elder-care workers in the United States. Because their wages as elder-care workers in the United States were so low, and because their work experiences have given them a sense of what an aged future in the United States might look like, they seek to retire back to Ghana, where they can live on their Social Security payments from the US government. Coe considers the fact that they cannot grow old in the United States to be an example of social and structural exclusion in the contemporary neoliberal environment. However, the aging migrants themselves frame their choices around the plight of the aged in the United States, a situation made visible by their employment in elder care. Mullings examines similar issues with her case study of older Caribbean women living in Canada, who were, like the Ghanaian migrants in Coe's study, working in low-paid jobs and sustaining family members back home through remittances. Now aged, they are in ill health and struggle financially, yet continue to contribute to communities in Canada and the Caribbean through making financial contributions to family and community, volunteering their time, and being active in their religious organizations. Unlike the Ghanaian migrants documented by Coe, they have remained in the country of migration rather than returning home as they thought they

would do. Like Coe, Mullings examines their situation as a sign of their exclusion and marginalization in Canada, using critical race feminism and counter-
stories as analytic underpinnings for her arguments.

Finally, Dossa's chapter brings us to the process of dying, an important
but challenging aspect of life to study. Her study, focusing on Ismaili Muslim
migrants in palliative care centers in Canada, argues that the end of life is a
highly significant time for kin work, in two ways. One, children drop their busy
lives to care for the dying, and two, the lifetime kin work of the dying person
is acknowledged and made visible by those around them. Like Yarris and Baldassar, Dossa considers kin work broadly as including memorializing efforts
through the recordings of religious songs and teaching the significance of prayer
and sacred places to young people. However, such kin work in palliative care
centers is mediated by the power of the biomedical model, which considers
the dying person to be an individual rather than embedded in social relations,
and by the institutional setting, which renders their cultural practices uncom-
fortably visible in a public space. Dossa imagines how palliative care might be
transformed and informed by attentiveness to what might seem insubstantial
and fleeting, such as food, photographs, and music, but which help kin connect
to one another, acknowledge the significance and status of the dying person,
and create memories across the generations.

The chapters in this volume examine the dynamics and tensions of aging
within the context of state policies, kin relationships, labor markets, and biomedical institutions as these unfold transnationally. In the process, we focus
on what is overlooked: the routine activities of aging people. In her research on
Persian female migrants in Australia, Deirdre Conlon (2011) argues that everyday practices of embroidery and cooking enfold memories of trauma. Such
practices, she notes, are bodies of knowledge that are continuously regenerated through daily actions. In a similar vein, Daniel Miller (2008) observes that
homely things help us to unravel people's embodied experiences. He puts it
this way: "Surely if we can learn to listen to these things, we have access to an
authentic other voice" (2). The chapters in this volume attend to the voices of
aging men and women (and their relatives) and the care practices that sustain
them and others as a way of gaining insight into how transnational families are
coping with the pressures of family regeneration in an era of austerity.

Aging, Globalization, and Transnational Families

Older people's kin work contributions and demands have become increasingly
significant to their families and communities because today families are under
pressure from the changing conditions of capitalism and declining state support for families. Saskia Sassen (2014) argues that in the contemporary world,

companies' profits depend less on workers' labor and consumption and more on resource extraction. This new dynamic has implications for the further fraying of the social contract with workers and their families, in which states and markets are becoming less invested in the education of the labor force and the provision of social services.

Some families respond to these pressures and strains by migrating. In other words, they make use of the differing political, social, and economic conditions of multiple countries to enable their survival. Living transnationally, they can use the resources available in various locations. For example, young and middle-aged adults may migrate, leaving behind their older relatives and children to live in better housing or attend better schools than they could afford in the country of migration. Older migrants may decide to retire to their country of origin, or another country altogether, to stretch their retirement savings further in a place with a lower cost of living or more kin support. Paul Kennedy and Victor Roudometof note, "Many transnational communities have been born out of the experience of social injustices, global inequalities, and chronic insecurities. Global economic restructuring, the post-1989 capitalistic boom and the ascendancy of neoliberal economic policies have further accentuated such experiences" (2002, 4). Sassen considers transnational migration to be evidence for the new dynamics of expulsion, in which poorer states are dependent on resource extraction and migrants' remittances. Restrictive immigration policies—which limit the entry of unskilled workers, the non-rich, and the aged—are also a significant part of the new politics of exclusion and inequality.

Another response to the shifting dynamics of capitalism and state policies is that families rely increasingly on the entrustments and reciprocities available to them through their kin networks, because they cannot survive on their wages. In particular, as the chapters in this volume show, in many countries, the parents of young children cannot pay the market rate for childcare because of their low wages and insecure employment. Because entrustment has a different kind of logic than wage labor or state benefits, families can use reciprocal relations to create a safety net for themselves when the market and state fail them. For instance, working parents turn to their own parents to provide unpaid childcare, whether in the country of origin or the country of migration, as several of the chapters in this volume illustrate. Grandmothers are often seen as particularly suited for this role, as part of the assignment of tasks to various kin members known as kin-scription. Another example of the way that people rely on kin to mitigate the failures of the labor market and state disbursements is that they may decide to return to their homeland to rely on reciprocal relationships available there (Coe, this volume). The uncertainty of pension payments may lead older adults to depend on their adult children instead (Deneva, this volume; Mullings, this volume). Yet all these sources of support are precarious and anxiety producing. The need to maintain connections across scattered family members and to the homeland—as part of the diverse ecology available for family sustenance—also speaks to the significance of the memorializing and homemaking work of the aged in keeping these connections across time and space active in the present (Baldassar, this volume; Dossa, this volume; Yarris, this volume). The contributions and demands of older adults thus are central to the survival and regeneration of families in contexts of migration.

The social roles and daily activities of older men and women tell us how globalization affects the intimate sphere of family life and individual life courses. Aging trajectories and the perception of what it means to be old are changing. As several of the chapters illustrate, because of changing social, economic, and political processes, older people are not always able to perform their socially expected roles as "good grandmothers" or "respected elders." Furthermore, middle-aged adults also feel inadequate in their roles as "dutiful daughters" (Khan and Koyabashi, this volume) or loving mothers (Raffety, this volume). Employment, retirement, and illness trajectories are not always easy to match with others' timing of fertility, employment, and schooling. Social inequalities in the wider world may create new social inequalities in family life, in which older adults suffer neglect, become dependent, or are socially marginal within their families. Thus, these chapters speak to the tensions and social inequalities within families and for the aged that the new politics of structural exclusion generate. Yet we also witness the enormous creativity and vitality of older adults as they seek to make themselves socially visible and valuable in the contexts they find meaningful, as the chapter by Raffety in particular illustrates. Older adults are shaping the world around them through their kin work and transforming the meaning of what it means to be old, through their "scraps, memories, and everyday realities."

NOTES

1. The notion of cultural projects comes from Sherry B. Ortner (2006).
2. Experimental field studies of discrimination in labor markets in Sweden and Spain show that younger workers are preferred (Ahmed, Andersson, and Hammerstedt 2012; Rocío, Escot, and Fernández-Cornejo 2011). But Jessica Greenberg and Andrea Muhlebach (2007) note that in Italy, older workers were increasingly preferred as the intergenerational contract shifted and as flexible, part-time work became more common.
3. Loosely translated by the author.
4. The accuracy of these statements about the dire state of Social Security has been challenged.

PART ONE

The Kin-scription of Older People into Care

1

Flexible Kin Work, Flexible Migration

Aging Migrants Caught between Productive and Reproductive Labor in the European Union

NEDA DENEVA

This chapter is concerned with the interplay between productive and reproductive labor performed by aging carers migrating within the European Union. It analyzes the ways in which this interplay is reconfigured in the context of migration and the ways in which this reconfiguration repositions aging carers as citizens and workers. Current labor regimes and freedom of movement in the European Union have enabled an intensification of short-term, semiseasonal labor migrations, which in turn has triggered a circulation of kin members performing kin work involving both productive and reproductive labor. This intensified migration has resulted in reconfigurations in kin relations and transformations in care work by creating new expectations and responsibilities.

The kin work of the aging is intergenerational, involving different types of care for children and grandchildren. The main carers are grandparents, and more specifically grandmothers, who fit the category of the young-old.[1] They are forty-five to fifty-five years old and are still considered of active working age, while simultaneously having care obligations for both their own elderly parents and their still young grandchildren. Employing a culturally sensitive and relational approach, I define them through their social age and their position in a care network, rather than by their biological age.[2] This definition allows me to use a generational perspective—that of the so-called sandwich generation[3]—to analyze the effect of care obligations. In this sense, social age groups overlap with generations defined through care commitments.[4]

In this chapter I analyze the experiences of transnational young-old carers in two cases of low-skilled migration from rural regions of Bulgaria—Bulgarian Muslims from the Gotse Delchev region in the southwest and Bulgarian Roma from the region of Shumen in the northeast—to other EU (European Union) countries—Spain and Germany/the Netherlands respectively. My focus is on the individual autonomy of young-old women who are simultaneously grandmothers and daughters-in-law and who are pressed to assume the role of carers for both the generation of their grandchildren and the generation of their own parents. Drawing on the experiences of young-old carers, I trace two types of newly emerging tensions: (1) the loss of access to social entitlements (social welfare) replaced by a new form of kin reciprocity (kinfare) in the case of the Bulgarian Muslims and (2) tensions between productive labor (financial autonomy) and reproductive labor (care work) in the case of the Bulgarian Roma.

The migration processes I describe here are part of two types of familial projects (Ortner 2006). In the first case, family members migrate together in an attempt to sustain both the family and the ideal of the so-called normal family that shares the same home. In the second case, family members focus on reproducing a family scattered across borders by providing both care and financial support. In both cases productive and reproductive labor are put in tension for the young-old who migrate back and forth in their efforts to sustain the reproduction of the family. Based on these insights, I argue that the migration of individual workers is not an individual enterprise, as EU policies suggest. Rather, migration is enabled and sustained by the reproductive labor of a number of interconnected agents in the migration process.[5] Both familial projects are built on transnationalized kin relations, which affect the dynamics between productive and reproductive labor for different kin members. In order to understand migratory decisions, we need to think of these mobilities as part of a common project of family reproduction, rather than as individual trajectories and experiences.[6] Considering the members of a transnational family as part of a single social field makes one appreciate the uneven effects of migration projects on these different members. Their different positioning reveals new inequalities and dependencies created by migration as well as the reinforcement of old ones. The generation of young-old carers becomes vulnerable by an acute repositioning in which their autonomy is challenged in at least three respects: by new inequalities between kin, by exclusion from the labor market, and by decreased access to social rights.

Care, Age, and Citizenship in Transnational Family Projects

For a long time, the migration literature has only looked at female migrants as wives and mothers and thus conceptualized them as followers and dependents and as unproductive, isolated, illiterate, and ignorant (Morokvasic 1983, 16). In more recent decades, migration scholars have challenged this perception and considered female migrants to be autonomous actors in dynamic migration processes. The central role of female migrants in the feminizing global labor market received special attention with a an emphasis on care work beginning in the last decade (e.g., Andall 2000; B. Anderson 2000; Hochschild 2003; Hondagneu-Sotelo 2007; Hondagneu-Sotelo and Avila 1997; Lutz 2010; Morokvasic 1983, 2004; Sassen 2000; Yeates 2009). In these studies, women are at the center of the migration process and are conceived as triggers of migration streams, breadwinners, and senders of remittances, rather than followers and dependents. I seek to complicate this dichotomy by focusing on the active role of female migrants as carers who provide reproductive labor in a migration model that is centered on the family. I found that older female migrants are neither the active trigger of migration nor the passive follower, but rather an indispensable agent in a familial migration project that depends on a complex distribution of productive and reproductive labor.

To understand these transnational carers, we need to look at the global transformation of care regimes in relation to migration and age. One way of approaching this topic is through the category of left-behind parents of younger migrants and the tensions that arise from renegotiated care arrangements and intergenerational reciprocity (Baldassar 2007; Baldock 2000, 2003; Mazzucato 2008a; Pyle 2006; van der Geest, Mul, and Vermeulen 2004). The concept of the care drain (Hochschild 2003) further enriches the analysis. Care drain refers to the phenomenon of immigrant young women providing paid care work in wealthier countries while leaving behind their own families and children. Other female kin usually fill this gap by creating a global care chain (Chamberlain 1997; Lutz 2007; Parreñas 2001). In these new care arrangements, aging people can be receivers of care performed by migrants (Andall 2000) or carers themselves for children left behind (Olwig 1999) or for children and older people in the receiving country. What is absent from this range of possibilities, however, is the category of aging migrants moving between geographical and institutional localities to provide care for different members of their own families. By doing so, they move the care chain geographically. This movement creates new types of tensions in their own lives and in their relations with dispersed kin.

Like most of the other contributors to this volume, I am convinced that the focus on kin work through an intergenerational perspective—which involves multidimentional relations of care and financial support—is necessary in order to fully understand how migration triggers ruptures in people's lives (see Dossa and Coe, this volume). Furthermore, temporality—both in terms of the life course and of future expectations and redefined reciprocities—is central for this chapter, as it is for most of the other chapters in this volume.

Thinking of women and elderly people in their role as carers requires us to further frame this issue through the globalization of kinship. The concepts of the transnational family (Bryceson and Vuorela 2002), the transnational domestic sphere (Gardner and Grillo 2002), global kin networks (Olwig 2002), and global house holding (Peterson 2010) emphasize that families are not discrete geographically or state-bound entities, but can be maintained across time and space. This transnational dispersal involves, however, the (re)negotiation of commitments, reciprocity, and duty, and practical mechanisms and strategies that are necessary for the reproduction of the family. In Glenn's (1992) broad definition, reproductive labor includes activities that maintain people both on a daily basis and intergenerationally, such as caring for children and adults, preserving community and family ties, and performing household tasks. In this sense, the transnationalization of families creates reproductive care chains in which carers involved in kin work are engaged in transnational mobilities themselves (see Kofman 2012).

The care-triggered mobility of young-old grandmothers from Bulgaria evolves in the particular context of EU migration and citizenship regimes. The role of migration policies and regimes, the inequalities in the global labor market, and the neoliberal restructuring of welfare regimes are all systematically producing transnational families and reconfiguring intergenerational relations, an issue also discussed by other authors in this volume (see Coe, Raffety, Zhou, all in this volume). Freedom of movement in the European Union has enabled the more intense mobility of young-old carers since 2007 when Bulgaria became an EU-member state. At the same time, the analysis of care-triggered migration of the aged reveals the heterogeneity of EU citizenship, in which different subcategories of internal migrants have access to different types of rights. Hence, they experience their mobility in different ways, facing different levels of exclusion. EU citizenship, conceived above all as enabling the circulation of productive labor, favors an understanding of the citizen as a worker (Hancock 1999). Social rights for EU migrants are not universal, but are conditional, and privilege those who are workers. Furthermore, the privileging of workers relies on a narrow conception of work as regular, full-time paid employment, which excludes a large number of workers engaged in part-time work, care work, nonstandard forms of employment, and informal employment.[7] The connection between access to welfare entitlements and regular full-time employment affects people who move as part of a male breadwinner family or work in irregular or part-time jobs, making them more vulnerable (Ackers 1998, 2004; Ackers and Dwyer 2002; McGlynn 2000, 2001; Stychin 2000). This conception of EU citizenship assumes an individualistic view of the citizen as an autonomous agent and worker, without acknowledging the need for unpaid reproductive labor performed by kin. This assumption renders the social citizenship of wives and aging kin members indirect, derivative, and relational, placing them in a position of dependent individuals, deepening patriarchal power relations and reinforcing kin reciprocity.

In order to understand the ruptures and reconfigurations that mobile aging carers experience in this context, I draw on ethnographic material from two periods of research in two different migrant communities. The case of the Bulgarian Muslims is based on extended ethnographic research for my dissertation, conducted translocally between 2007 and 2009 in Bulgaria and in Spain, with subsequent shorter research trips. The case of the Bulgarian Roma is based on ongoing qualitative research since the summer of 2013 and extending into the fall of 2014 in the region of Shumen, Bulgaria. I look at daily care arrangements, the everyday ruptures that these new arrangements trigger, and the way people make sense of their practices and repositioning. Combining research on discourses and practices, I employ methods that include life stories, extended semi-structured interviews, and informal conversations. I have participated in social and family events, alongside everyday activities, like walks in the park, shopping trips, picking up and dropping off children at school, and other daily routines.

In what follows, I trace two types of transnational kin work performed by aging carers, aiming to illustrate the various strategies crafted to deal with the gaps that migration causes in care arrangements. These new arrangements trigger tensions and ruptures in intergenerational relations and in the position of the young-old as autonomous individuals, both economically and in terms of social welfare. In the first case, migration leads to transformations in intergenerational relations and care arrangements and at the same time in the aging carer's access to social entitlements. These two transformations create new types of kin dependencies and trigger new insecurities about the future. In the second case, the tension is more clearly one between the productive and reproductive labor of the aging carer who has to provide care for the reproduction of the younger generation's family and financial support for themselves and other kin members through productive labor. Intense mobility and the specifics of available work in different locations (i.e., the lack of formal work opportunities for Bulgarian Muslim aging women in Spain, and the lack of decent work opportunities for Bulgarian Roma women in Bulgaria) put these two obligations in conflict. In both cases, what is at stake is the autonomy of the carers who see their rights and financial independence limited by a move toward kin reliance and new reciprocities. I have previously called this shift a move to "kinfare" (Deneva 2012).

Bulgaria is an Eastern European country whose social security system and labor market underwent major transformations since the collapse of state socialism. The position of the socialist woman was that of an individual enjoying social security by virtue of her position as a worker and as a socialist citizen. Even for younger women who might not have personally experienced universal access to employment and the security of welfare, the obligations and entitlements of previous generations functioned as the standard against which to measure present conditions. In this sense, the definition of work is historically constructed, even for younger generations. Confinement solely to reproductive labor through care and kin making is not a familiar practice for generations of working-class women in Bulgaria. They consider reliance on a male kin member like a husband or son for present and future financial support a rupture in their life trajectories, preferring personal income from productive labor and/or welfare entitlements. Such reliance affects the way these women experience their relationship with and obligations to kin.

The first massive emigration waves from Bulgaria started after the demise of state socialism in 1989. Due to liberalized border visa regimes, political instability, and economic transformations leading to high unemployment and inflation, the number of Bulgarian emigrants by 2007 reached, according to different sources, between 600,000 and one million or up to 12 percent of the population. Although there is no consensus on the periodization of the different migration waves, scholars have roughly divided it into four periods, which reflect policy changes in the migration regimes of destination countries vis-à-vis Bulgarian citizens, rather than solely political and economic conditions in Bulgaria (Jileva 2002; Mancheva 2011; Markova 2010). First, the first few years after 1989 were marked by early political emigration by Bulgarian Turks into Turkey, and other Bulgarian citizens into the West, asking for political asylum. In the second period from the mid-1990s until 2001, the economic crisis in Bulgaria caused migration in the context of tightening immigration controls and strict visa regimes in Western European countries and the United States. The third period from 2001 to 2007 is the pre-EU accession period, which witnessed a liberalization of mobility in the European Union (visa-free travel allowed for up to three months), which intensified migration significantly. It is in this period that both the Bulgarian Muslims and the Bulgarian Roma described in this chapter started migrating on a larger scale into Western Europe, predominantly relying on networks of kin and covillagers, and thus forming a chain-migration pattern. The fourth period is the post-2007 EU membership of Bulgaria and involves the free movement of citizens and the gradual lifting of labor market restrictions. This period witnessed initially high numbers of migration until 2009, when the financial crisis affected migration.

Both cases take place in the context of low-skilled, poverty-driven labor migration within the European Union, which allows mobility and flexibility. However, there are variations within this type of mobility depending on the opportunities for employment, labor relations, and the availability of care and carers. Thus, the ruptures and transformations taking place vary in both cases. Yet, the most vulnerable and most negatively affected in both cases are the young-old carers.

A Move from Welfare to Kinfare: The Case of Zaira

Zaira is a Bulgarian Muslim migrant torn between care obligations to her father-in-law in Bulgaria, her son's children in Spain, and her daughter's children in Spain. In her complicated care network, there is little space for her to act as a worker and as a full-fledged participant in Bulgaria's welfare system. Her care obligations are spread geographically and lead to a transgression of the ideal patrilocal care regimes of the community. By including her daughter's family in her reproductive labor, Zaira reconfigures kin relations that now lead to new insecurities about her future. At the same time, her devotion to reproductive labor is accompanied by stepping out of her position as a worker who, by means of her active participation in the workforce, also had access to employment-based welfare—a retirement plan, free health care, and unemployment benefits. As a result, her future and present support depends solely on her kin.

Zaira's story develops in the context of Bulgarian Muslim migration to Spain. She comes from a village in the Western Rhodopi mountains where more than half of the inhabitants have migrated to the Spanish region of Navarra. Their migration picked up after 2001, when Schengen visa restrictions were lifted for Bulgarian citizens, and further intensified after 2007 when Bulgaria became an EU-member state. EU freedom of mobility allowed for more short-term visits and movement not motivated by employment, especially by the kin of initial labor migrants. Typically, Bulgarian Muslims migrated to Spain in clusters in a network-based chain migration, thus re-creating village relations, including social relations of support, celebrations, and everyday interactions in new localities in Spain. Intergenerational care arrangements were also reproduced, but only at first sight.

The instigators of this migration were young male workers who found jobs in construction and as truck drivers in Spain before the 2008 economic crisis and have mostly kept their positions until now. Once a man settled into a job, his wife and children would arrive (Deneva 2013). Women thus came to Spain in a second wave in their capacity as mothers and wives joining their husbands. While men often have full-time jobs, even if in the informal sector and under flexible conditions, the majority of the young women work in precarious part-time employment, mostly in domestic service and catering jobs. Ironically, such part-time and odd jobs interfere with caring for the children, since working hours and shifts in these sectors extend beyond nursery and school hours. At the same time, the income of a sole working man is not enough to support the whole family, so young women are financially pressured to engage in at least part-time work. Thus, the reproduction of the young family in Spain requires external support for care work. This need gradually triggered a third stage of

migratory movements: the arrival of aging carers. Young migrants with children started inviting their parents, the young old, to Spain in moments of care
crisis—during school vacations, on the occasions of short-term intense employment of younger women, or around the birth of a new child—to provide assistance with child-rearing and household activities, initially for limited periods of
time but gradually extending to longer periods.

In this migration pattern where members of a family migrate in consecu-
tive waves, migration does not appear to disrupt the family fabric, but instead
restores the kin support network, which allows the family to be reproduced
in Spain. One might conclude that the overall well-being of the family unit is
improved. Contrast it with the migratory practice of *gourbet*, where lone Balkan
male temporary migrants were away from their families for extended periods
of time. Or with the exclusively female care work migration, widespread among
middle-aged women who support their children and husbands back home with
remittances. On the contrary, the current type of migration aims to reinforce
kinship relations and reproduce the village community, while increasing the
family's economic prospects and giving them access to social entitlements that
they lack at home. Indeed, on the streets of Tafalla, one would often see whole
migrant families strolling together. Living arrangements for most migrants
were organized along the lines of the nuclear family and a care-taking grandparent. When members of the nuclear family were divided spatially, this was
only a transitional stage before all would be reunited in one place, usually in
Spain. However, a closer look uncovers the cracks in this picture of re-created
social relations.

Whereas young people considered their migration long term from the out-
set, transnational aging carers initially conceived of their mobility as temporary
and strictly oriented to the care needs of their family, even though their migrations have often become extended as well. Typically, it was women who arrived
first for short periods of time to solve a particular care crisis. After a few visits,
their husbands might also join them, trying to find a temporary job as day laborers in agriculture or construction. At times, their migration became permanent
with both elderly parents settling in Spain. Alternatively, carers might keep
coming for short periods every few months to provide temporary care relief
while the daughter worked in a temporary position, for school holidays, or at
the birth of a new baby. In both scenarios, elderly migrants are in Spain as a
subsidiary group for the main purpose of providing care work.[8] Although aging
people's mobility reconstituted the care support network, it disrupted their own
employment and social benefits status.

In Bulgaria, women in the Rhodopi region are mainly employed in sewing
factories and workshops. On the side, many elderly women also used to grow
tobacco for subsidiary income and often owned a cow for the home use and

sale of dairy products. Before her migration, Zaira worked in a sewing factory in addition to growing tobacco over the summer. Before 1992, she worked in a local factory. Soon after most of the industry in the region was privatized and closed down, Greek entrepreneurs arrived to set up small sewing workshops employing women under exploitative conditions. At the time I met Zaira, conditions had improved: workers received the minimum salary and had regular employment contracts with social benefits included.

Zaira had a small garden next to her house used for subsistence agriculture and owned a cow. Her daughter-in-law used to help her with the tobacco and the cow before she migrated to Spain. Once the young family left, Zaira's daughter assisted with the tobacco for one summer, before she herself went to Spain. Zaira could not manage the tobacco fields alone and quit.[9] A similar pattern occurred in many other families not only due to the unfavorable price of tobacco, but also because of disruptions to work patterns caused by the migration of the younger generation. Zaira lost her second source of additional income, her cow, when her son summoned her to Spain to assist with his newborn baby. She had to sell the cow because she was not able to take care of it or leave it with anyone during the two months she was away.

Zaira's experience of losing these two sources of income was typical for most elderly women with migrant kin. After her first trip to Spain in the summer of 2006 came another trip the following spring, when her daughter-in-law found a fixed-term substitute full-time job in a restaurant and she and her son needed support with their nine-month-old baby. In the meantime, Zaira's daughter, who lived in the same small town in Spain, gave birth, and asked Zaira to extend her stay to assist her. Zaira agreed, moving to her daughter's house in a nearby neighborhood, while simultaneously trying to assist her son's family with childcare by dropping off and picking up the older two children from school every day.

The stay with her daughter's family caused two types of tensions in Zaira's life. First, she had to combine care work for her son's and for her daughter's family, which disrupted ideal care regimes of the patrilocal tradition where care work flows between a son and his parents. This opened a space for moral critique from other kin members and covillagers. Had this situation happened in the village, Zaira would have been able to remain living in her son's house and taking care of his children, while simultaneously providing childcare for her daughter's son. Moving to her daughter's house highlighted that she was providing kin work proper to her daughter and that it was her daughter whom she was supporting rather than her son. Zaira's experience of being stretched between two young families was quite common. Since grandparents were not themselves settled in Spain on a permanent basis, their visits always included staying in one of their children's houses. Migration disrupted everyday geographies and living patterns, which in turn aggravated the difficulties of balancing new care arrangements and responsibilities to the younger generations.

Furthermore, this extended period of stay in Spain, which followed the previous interruption, changed Zaira's employment position in the sewing factory. She took long periods of unpaid leave to be able to travel. In these periods, her employment contract was interrupted, which also disrupted her welfare contributions. Recovering her access to free health care after her leave, for example, meant paying retrospectively for at least six months[10] after going through administrative hurdles in the nearby town, a complication that Zaira decided to forgo, deciding instead to pay the full cost of health care when she needed it. Over the next year, she went back to Spain two more times. Eventually her husband also joined her and found a job in a construction company where their son also worked. When her husband found employment in Spain, Zaira quit her job in the sewing factory altogether and moved to Spain for an indefinite period. Quitting her job at the age of fifty-three excluded her from the regular labor market in Bulgaria, suspended her length of service early, having already been interrupted several times over the previous two years, and stopped any further participation in the welfare system, which was based on her employment contribution payments. In this way, her care-triggered migration to Spain deprived Zaira of employment-based welfare services in Bulgaria. There was also no compensation for her deprivation: a full welfare package was not open to her as a citizen of the European Union, because she was not formally employed in Spain.

Zaira had to change her plan of permanently moving to Spain several times. Once, she had to go back for an emergency concerning her mother-in-law, who had broken a leg and needed assistance. Although Zaira was not the correct daughter-in-law responsible for caring for the generation of the old-old, being married to the middle son, rather than the youngest, she still had to go because that daughter-in-law was also in Spain, taking care of the baby of her own son. The extended family considered her circumstances more pressing than Zaira's. Such rearrangements of care responsibilities were necessary because of the geographical distance and the dispersal of the kin. But these rearrangements disturbed different kin members who had to reconsider future reciprocity.

During Zaira's stay in Bulgaria, her son was constantly complaining that his own family needed her to return to Spain. At the time, his wife was working full-time in a nursing home and had to ask for unpaid leave in her mother-in-law's absence in order to handle childcare. The daughter-in-law commented that she and her husband supported her mother-in-law in Spain because of the care she provides, but they had to be able to rely on her. This direct financial dependency, which required full-time devotion to care work only in relation to one generation and one nuclear family, created more static relations and limited sets of possibilities. Migration limited the dynamism of having multiple, diverse resources like employment, additional means of income like tobacco and a cow, and kin work toward multiple relatives in different households.

Zaira's case was common for most young-old women who had started to migrate intensively for the purpose of providing care. The emphasis on their reproductive role leads to a reconfiguration of their position as autonomous economic agents and citizens entitled to welfare. The younger generation temporarily balanced these women's loss of autonomy by providing financial support. In this respect, kin work was two directional. The young-old carers had to stop relying on employment-based welfare and had to replace it with reliance on kin.

Kin reciprocity became the sole security strategy for migrant aging women. In this sense, kinfare substituted for welfare (see Deneva 2012). However, the move from productive to reproductive labor and from welfare to kinfare was not smooth, mostly due to the transformations in ideal care regimes relying on patriarchal arrangements between sons and their parents. The involvement of the daughters' families in care arrangements destabilized certainty in future reciprocity. Zaira shared with me her concerns of who is going to support her in the future, if she is spreading her assistance now between multiple children. By doing so, she was changing accepted patterns of reciprocity in which the youngest son inherits the house and lives in it with his family, taking care of his parents. However, the new geographic scattering of adult children across borders put this scheme in jeopardy.

Zaira explicitly worried about the future, especially in regard to health problems, looking at the experiences of her peers who got sick. There were two cases of aging migrant women who needed serious surgery for heart conditions and cancer and had to go back to Bulgaria and pay out-of-pocket for medical treatments, which were quite expensive. In both cases, there was family tension about who would cover the expenses for their mother. Zaira worried that if something similar happened to her, she would not know whom to ask for support, and that her children might also get into conflict with one another. The other worry was related to her future pension. Because of her shortened length of service, her potential retirement pension would only be minimal, which at present is certainly not enough to live on, even in a Bulgarian village. Relying solely on kinfare through reciprocity seemed insecure, after so many years of future planning to retire as a worker. Her transformation from a worker with care obligations into a full-time carer triggered both present and future insecurities, and new dependencies on her family.

Changed kin relations raise questions about future reciprocity. At the same time, reciprocity remains the only strategy for the future. Any individual autonomy on the part of aging women has been lost for the sake of the reproduction of the family. Most elderly women are engaged in one way or another in such novel care arrangements. The geographic distance makes it impossible to combine productive labor with care work and leads to new vulnerabilities for most. In this way, the migration of the younger generation, aimed at improvement of their own economic position made possible by the EU freedom of mobility and open labor markets, reconfigures the position of aging carers within the structure of the kin relations, and as workers and citizens.

Caught between Productive and Reproductive Labor: The Case of Sylvia

Sylvia is a Bulgarian Roma migrant in the Netherlands expected to provide financial support through remittances to her daughter's young family and to be present in Bulgaria to perform care obligations toward her son's son, who is just about to start school. She is torn between these two types of obligations, both framed morally as her responsibility toward the family. In this sense, both the financial provision and the care work constitute kin work. Productive and reproductive labor overlap and are interrelated. However, the mobility of kin members places these kin obligations in conflict. Unlike Zaira, Sylvia had trouble finding work in Bulgaria, and provides financially for herself and her daughter as a labor migrant in the Netherlands. At the same time, she is expected to provide care for her grandson in Bulgaria and rely solely on the financial help of her son.

The context in which this case evolves is slightly different from Zaira's. The type of migration is still low skilled and within the European Union. Nonetheless, access to secure and longer-term employment, abroad and in Bulgaria, is more limited than for Bulgarian Muslims for these reasons in varying degrees: (1) regional differences in terms of agriculture and industry; (2) factors like lack of landownership and fewer resources in general, typical situations for the rural Roma population; (3) prevalent ethnic discrimination and racism disrupting access to the labor market. Employment in this area of Bulgaria, when available at all, is precarious and exclusively informal, involving herb picking paid per piece, agricultural day labor, or work in small factories available for a limited number of workers. In Bulgaria, none of the families could afford to support themselves exclusively through work, but were reliant on remittances and meager welfare benefits. They lived in stark poverty with many people crammed in one-room houses, without running water or connection to a sewage system. Thus, the scarcity of work affects migration patterns. Roma migrants from the region of Shumen mostly migrate to the Netherlands, Germany, and Belgium, relying on relations with established Turkish migrants in these countries. For the purpose of this chapter, I will only focus on the situation of those migrants engaged in highly precarious and short-term, informal labor. Although there are cases of people who managed to establish themselves and their families abroad, the majority of migrants from the region travel back and forth, staying in one country for only a few months. Often, they spend their summer months in Bulgaria. When abroad, their accommodation patterns are unstable: they rent rooms per week, or even pay per bed in overcrowded bedrooms. When whole families live together, they usually share crowded flats, at times with temporary lodgers who are strangers.

The kind of work available to the Roma in the Netherlands is highly precarious: informal and short term, for which they are paid per week or per piece. Men work on small construction sites, in Turkish fast food shops, or on the street, playing music. The women work as street newspaper vendors,[11] domestic cleaners, factory workers, and field hands. The common thread between all these arrangements is that the work is informal, flexible, insecure, and very poorly paid. In such circumstances, settling down with children is a much more complicated endeavor.

The decision of many parents is to leave their children behind in Bulgaria. In those cases where children have accompanied their parents for certain periods, they are usually sent home permanently by the time they are ready to start school at six or seven years old. Parents need a full-time carer for the children during their migratory absences. These are usually the grandparents, most commonly the grandmother. While the parents go back and forth for short periods, making a living by combining different labor opportunities in two or three locations, the grandparents' home becomes that of their grandchildren.

Sylvia belongs to the Turkish-speaking Roma community in a village in Bulgaria's northeast. She speaks Bulgarian, Turkish, and Romani. She is forty-eight years old and has graduated from eighth grade, the minimum mandatory level of education. At the age of sixteen, she started working in a glass factory not far from the village where she used to live with her parents. Sylvia worked there for eight years, until she was made redundant in one of the waves of factory restructuring after the collapse of state socialism in 1989. She has three children. When we spoke in the summer of 2013, the eldest son was twenty-nine years old, the daughter was twenty-six, and another son had just turned nineteen and gotten married. Sylvia worked occasionally in agriculture after the factory closed down, but her family was barely getting by since her husband also had a hard time finding regular work. Employment was informal and poorly paid, and did not provide enough income to support her family even though she shared a household with her parents-in-law. After the relaxation of mobility for Bulgarian citizens in the European Union in 2001, both Sylvia and her husband went to work in the Netherlands, where they got separated. Their children remained with Sylvia's mother in Bulgaria, the youngest then eight years old. Sylvia was sending remittances and barely making ends meet in the Netherlands.

Her job there was in a mushroom factory, where she worked without a formal labor contract. Her income depended on the length of shifts pegged to the daily growth of the mushrooms. She slept in shared rooms paying per bed per week, ready to leave whenever she ran out of money. When her youngest son turned thirteen, he started getting into trouble and his grandmother could not control him anymore. Sylvia came back to Bulgaria for a few months, but realized that she could not find any employment there and soon took her adolescent son with her to the Netherlands. There, they both worked in the mushroom factory for the same employer. She continued to send money to her two other children. A year later, her eldest son, who was then twenty-four years old, came to work in the Netherlands. He soon brought his wife and baby. Sylvia suddenly had to choose between full-time work in the mushroom factory and assisting her son with the baby. The eldest son worked in a Turkish fast-food shop and his wife sold street newspapers. Through these two incomes, they could afford to rent a private room. Sylvia arranged with her boss to start working part-time, enabling her to take care of the baby. Her son's arrival to the Netherlands relieved Sylvia of the obligation to support him financially. Yet she continued sending small amounts of money to her mother and to her daughter who remained in the village and continued to support her still underage younger son. This arrangement lasted for several years, with Sylvia always living in a financially precarious situation.

When we first met in the village in 2013, her youngest son had just gotten married in Bulgaria. Her daughter and son-in-law migrated back and forth to the Netherlands and Germany for short-term jobs, but were barely making ends meet. Her eldest son and his wife had continued to work abroad, combining this with occasional prolonged stays in Bulgaria, when their income was not sufficient to cover their expenses. Sylvia was now settled in Bulgaria. She was living with her ill mother, taking care of her, and working in agriculture seasonally under very difficult conditions. A typical representative of the sandwich generation, Sylvia was torn between care for her grandchildren and for her own parents, although she was in her prime years of productive labor. However, the chief reason for Sylvia's return to Bulgaria was her grandson, the eldest son of her eldest son. When he was younger, his parents would take him with them to the Netherlands, where they relied on Sylvia for part-time support, and often traveled back to Bulgaria. Once he turned six years old though, his parents chose to send him back to Bulgaria. This meant a relocation for Sylvia as well, who had to stop working in the Netherlands and return to Bulgaria to care for her grandson.

The decision to send school-aged children back to Bulgaria is very common among the migrants and is conditioned by the particular structural conditions in which Roma labor migration occurs. For the Roma, the available labor opportunities are very unstable and precarious: informal employment with no contracts, short-term or piece work, low pay and exploitative conditions. This type of labor mobility is impermanent, and often comprised of brief intervals. Migrants combine their work in other countries with periods of work in Bulgaria where they engage in other short-term jobs. This particular pattern, which is rather different from the one of the Bulgarian Muslims described above, has to do with the limited resources at their disposal, the type of labor market that the Roma enter in Germany and the Netherlands, the intermediation of the Turkish middlemen, and the Roma's stigmatized social position in Bulgaria. In Bulgaria, they work in now-collapsed industries and agriculture without owning the land. In addition, the relaxed regimes of EU mobility allow for short-term circular mobility.

These irregular mobilities and labor practices affect the lives of all family members. The extreme mobility does not allow parents to settle down with their children in one geographical location for a long period. The instability turns out to be particularly problematic once children turn school age and parents are obliged by law to enroll them in school. There are examples of parents who attempted to settle abroad along with their children, only later to discover that they could not support the whole family. The end result was that parents sent their children back to the care of other relatives, most commonly grandparents. At the same time, the educational system in Bulgaria, like most educational systems, is nation-state bound and is a source of ruptures for transnational children (see Hamann and Zúñiga 2011). Once a child misses a year, reenrollment turns out to be extremely difficult. The results from a recent study (Mineva et al., forthcoming) demonstrate that many children in such situations had to reenroll at a lower grade and lose up to two years, due to the rigid bureaucratic procedures of the formal educational system.

This complicated picture—of low-skilled, poorly paid informal labor patterns; a highly flexible migration regime, involving EU freedom of mobility; a lack of available means of living at home; and rigid state educational policies—frames the decisions of mobile parents to leave their school-aged children at home. However, this decision creates new care arrangements that, more often than not, trigger major ruptures in the lives of the carers, as the case of Sylvia clearly shows. Once she returned to Bulgaria to take care of her grandchildren, she stopped being able to generate enough income to make a living for herself and her dependents. Two complications resulted: first, she stopped being able to financially support her daughter's family, a situation that triggered moral accusations and conflicts; second, she stopped being able to provide enough financial support for herself and became dependent on her son's remittances. In these circumstances, she was pressured to take any available work, like herb picking, agricultural day labor, or any other odd job that might come her way (Deneva 2015). Thus, Sylvia's return to Bulgaria to perform her obligations as a caring grandmother caused several ruptures. Her relations with her daughter had become tense, she became financially dependent on her elder son, and her own sense of autonomy was compromised. At the same time, she felt idle at an age in which she wanted, and was able, to be productive and generate her own income.

Unlike the case of the Bulgarian Muslim migrants, the tension here derives less from the loss of social rights and more from financial dependence. Given the marginal structural position of the Bulgarian Roma migrants, engaged in informal employment, access to social benefits is structurally limited from the onset (Deneva 2015). However, in both cases, migration of some kin members is made possible by others, who are engaged in kin making through care work. The ruptures are caused by the decoupling of productive and reproductive labor. In the case of the Bulgarian Muslims, the main aspect of kin work is care, which due to migration triggers disruptions in the carers' social citizenship; in the case of the Roma, kin work involves both care work and financial support. In this case, productive and reproductive labors overlap and come in conflict. This overlap triggers new expectations and reconfigurations of people's lives.

Conclusion

Drawing on two cases of aging carers engaged in complex mobility, I have presented how migration strains the balance between productive and reproductive labor and calls for a readjustment of care arrangements and kin relations. In this process, the members of the sandwich generation, the young-old, most commonly women, are the most vulnerable. They have to balance their obligations to different kin members (sons and daughters, grandchildren and aging parents) with their position as workers and participants in a welfare regime accruing rights through their paid employment in the formal sector, not through their care work. In both cases, the individual autonomy of these carers is at stake. Individual autonomy is often lost for the sake of the reproduction of the migrant family. By taking upon themselves the burden of kin work in a transnational family project, these carers experience ruptures in their present and future social and financial security.

Transnational migration not only triggers a reformulation of gender and intergenerational relations in the family. It also generates transformations in the realm of social citizenship entitlements and in access to work. Freedom of mobility within the European Union facilitates the transnational care practices of the young-old and gives them hope for their children's economic advancement. At the same time, the freedom of mobility disrupts their own social citizenship and financial independence, whether in Bulgaria or the country of migration, losing employment, welfare entitlements, and additional sources of income. Consequently, the trans-nationalization of the family affects the aging carers' autonomy and social citizenship, while allowing their children to acquire a more secure position abroad and to reproduce their own families.

The recent intensification of mobility also triggers a disrupted sense of home and belonging. The aging carers' role in the reproduction of the migrant family requires them to flexibly provide care for two different generations dispersed in two or more localities. It creates a conflict between productive and reproductive labor. What is at stake, however, is not only their present, but also their future, survival. The aging carers in both cases lose their autonomy and financial independence by stepping out of their role as workers and citizens with access to welfare, pensions, and health benefits by virtue of performing productive labor. Younger people are able to advance both their economic well-being and their social citizenship through migration, but only with the support of aging carers who lose their few guarantees in terms of employment and social security. The emphasis on family reproduction through care signifies a move from welfare to kinfare, in which kin reciprocity replaces state support and financial independence through one's own productive labor. Aging women, as the main providers of care across localities and states, fall into a particularly precarious position, risking any stability they had in Bulgaria, in the case of Bulgarian Muslims, or the financial independence they had abroad, in the case of the Bulgarian Roma, for the sake of fulfilling their kin work. Full dependency on the younger generation in the future along with the uncertainties of their present everyday lives creates new forms of gendered and intergenerational inequalities. Transformations in kinship intertwine with transformations in citizenship and individual autonomy for the young-old grandmothers—not only in the present but also in the future.

NOTES

1. This definition is based on Bernice L. Neugarten's (1974, 1996) distinction between the different stages of old age into young-old and old-old. The old-old in this context would be the parents of the young-old who are themselves in need of care.

2. For an analysis of the socially constructed and contextually sensitive transition from middle age to old age, see Gubrium, Holstein, and Buckholdt 1994; Hazan 1992; Laz 1998.

3. The term "sandwich generation" usually denotes middle-aged women who simultaneously work and provide care for both their still-dependent children and their aging parents. Here I expand this term to include the generation caring for grandchildren and aging parents.

4. Generation in this text refers to the narrow sense of a position within a family, which changes over a lifetime from grandchild to grandparent.

5. For alternative discussions of migration as a family project, see Fedyuk 2011; Kraler et al. 2011; Olwig 2007, 2012; Stephen 2007.

6. On migration as a family economic strategy see also Baldassar, this volume.

7. Informal work is one way to refer to a labor activity that is licit in every sense other than being registered or declared to the state for tax benefit purpose (see European Commission 1998; ILO 2002). It involves avoiding tax and benefit contributions both by the worker and by the employer, which deprives the worker from access to welfare based on employment (like unemployment benefits, a certain form of health insurance, or retirement plan, depending on the country), and from the protection of any labor codes and health and safety regulations. In addition, informal employment also makes workers vulnerable and more easily exploitable due to lack of any form of security of their pay and length of employment.

8. Any employment undertaken by the older men in this context is for very little money and is regarded as extra to help support the enlarged household rather than for personal needs.

9. Tobacco growing is considered a woman's job. Men usually do not participate on a regular basis, being engaged with other full-time activities in the summer months like stone tiling, construction, or forestry, in some cases away from the village.

10. As of March 2016, the regulation changed to paying all missed health insurance contributions retrospectively (up to five years) in order to restore one's health coverage rights.

11. Street papers are produced specifically for homeless and poor people in many countries around the world. They are sold at a small price (usually half the cover price) and then resold in public spaces (for more on this issue, see Cockburn 2013). More on one of the networks of street paper sellers can be found at: http://www.street-papers.org/about-us.

2

The New Aging Trajectories of Chinese Grandparents in Canada

YANQIU RACHEL ZHOU

Canada's policies on the sponsoring of parents and grandparents for immigration have tightened since the Conservative Party assumed power in 2008. Despite an eight-year-long waiting list, in 2011 the federal government announced a two-year freeze on permanent residency applications from the parents and grandparents of permanent residents and citizens (Elliott 2012). In 2014 it reopened the door a crack for older immigrants by accepting five thousand sponsorship applications under the new Parent and Grandparent Program, with its unprecedented stringent criteria for sponsoring relatives: that is, a higher and more stable family income and an increase of the sponsoring period from ten years to twenty (CBC News 2014). In the ensuing debate the deeper rationale for the policy changes became clear: older immigrants participate much less in the labor market and use the public health system much more (Gunter 2011). Describing older immigrants as "a burden on Canadian taxpayers" and their use of the social welfare systems as "an abuse of Canada's generosity," then Citizenship and Immigration Canada (CIC) Minister Jason Kenny could not have said it more bluntly: "If you think your parents may need to go on welfare in Canada, please don't sponsor them" (Fitzpatrick 2013, para. 16, ll. 1–2). This attitude, however, ignores immigrant families' frequent reliance on seniors for childcare and the variety of non-nuclear family arrangements among immigrants.

Neoliberal welfare restructuring has undermined the work of care in various ways that include the reduction of both the time available for care work and the state's capacity or willingness to provide care resources. When public care provision is inadequate or difficult to access, the traditional care burden of women who face work/family conflicts may be transferred onto paid care workers through the global care market, or onto their own family members—including elderly kin—through familial networks (Williams 2011; Yeates 2012; Zhou 2013). Since the 1990s the People's Republic of China (PRC) has become the premier source country of Canadian immigration. The majority of these immigrants hold a university degree and are often referred to as "skilled immigrants" (Li 2011). The recent influx of skilled immigrants from the PRC to major Canadian cities has been followed by the immigration of Chinese seniors, who work as housework helpers or, even, as primary caregivers in the homes of their immigrant children, who often are torn between reproductive labor and work/study. Despite occasional publicity of their plight—a heavy care work burden at home, economic dependence, family conflicts, social isolation, and health problems—in Chinese media in Canada (Chen 2006; Han 2005; Lang 2006), little has been written about the experiences of this elderly group.

Drawing on data from a larger empirical study of Chinese skilled immigrant families' transnational caregiving practices in Canada, this chapter explores the impact of adult children's immigration on their elderly parents' life trajectories. The findings of this study suggest that although those seniors' unprecedented mobility has helped to alleviate the childcare deficit experienced by their children as skilled immigrants in Canada, it has also had long-term effects on aging that are in contrast with seniors' own cultural expectations about, and individual preferences for, their later lives. Their adult children's emigration in China and their own participation in transnational care has disrupted the major aspects—such as intergenerational relation, filial piety, self-identity, and elder-care arrangement—of their movement into older age. Situating these seniors' experiences in the broader contexts of immigration, transnational family, and transnational care, this chapter contends that aging should no longer be understood as consisting solely of individuals' advancement into old age "in place" or in a domestic context. Aging is a dynamic, transnational process that intersects with intergenerational relationships, changing social roles of these seniors, and the effects of public policies—none of which is constrained by the geographic borders of a nation-state. The invisible incorporation of older Chinese immigrants into the global economy—in other words, through unpaid childcare—has also revealed the contradictions between Canada's immigration policy and care policy, and the effects of these policies beyond state borders and the nuclear family. The unpaid nature of grandparents' transnational caregiving and the state's failure to support immigrant families' mobilization of kin-based care from outside Canada evidence the multiple inequalities and exploitations (based on gender, age, migrant status, and geography) of care within families and between states. They also reflect the uneven effects of the restructuring of immigration and care regimes on individual and familial levels.

The Changing Context of Aging Research

Although research in general on older people in the context of international migration is modest in quantity, some progress at both the empirical and conceptual levels has prompted more attention in this area. Empirically, the issues around elder care in a transnational context have become salient both for international migrants whose parents were left behind in home countries and for migrant workers who are now themselves entering old age (Ammann and van Holten 2013; Baldassar, this volume; Baykara-Krumme 2013; Coe, this volume). Conceptually, older people are now viewed as members of transnational families or families maintaining ties across national borders, rather than solely as dependent on their adult immigrant children (Lunt 2009). According to Loretta Baldassar, Cora Vellecoop Baldock, and Raelene Wilding, the transnational family, as a new form of family, arises through "the exchange of care and support across distance and national borders" (2007, 14).

The endurance of familial ties across countries is the consequence of the autonomous choice of family members (including older ones) to maintain the family as an important traditional institution in which various sociocultural norms—kin keeping, generational reciprocity, elder care, cultural transference, and desired identity—continue, and in which resources—emotional support, help, care, and economic resources—are exchanged across generations (Baldassar, Baldock, and Wilding 2007; Lamb 2002; Lan 2002; Liu 2006; Mason 2004; Treas and Mazumdar 2004). From a critical perspective, however, the number of transnational households functioning as "cooperative units" indicates the importance of examining the macrostructural conditions that lead family members to live apart and that, in some cases, create new conflicts and inequality within families (Dreby and Adkins 2010). Transnational family arrangements, including care arrangements, are also the results of "stringent migration policies in migrant receiving countries that make it difficult for families to migrate together" (Mazzucato and Schans 2011, 704). The widely documented separation of migrant workers, including care workers, in wealthy countries from their families (including elderly parents) back home suggests that transnational families are systematically produced through various inequalities in the global labor market, border control policies, and access to social rights (Bernhard, Landolt, and Goldring 2009; Boccagni 2012; Dreby and Adkins 2010; Zentgraf and Chinchilla 2012). Immigrants' reliance on their transnational families for care and economic survival suggests that kinship or family, as a socioeconomic strategic unit, serves a flexible yet critical function in stabilizing or strengthening the family economy and in subsidizing labor migration in the face of these inequalities (Lomnitz 1977; Treas and Mazumdar 2004; Zhou 2013). In such cases, members—in particular, grandparents—of transnational families "act as collectives, strategizing to maximize economic gains given existing socio-economic and political restraints" (Dreby and Adkins 2010, 680). Yet such strategies may increase inequalities borne by the family as a whole, as well as by elderly family members.

Stressing the effects of social changes on people's lives, Glen H. Elder, Jr. (1994) identifies four central aspects: the relation between human lives and a changing society; the timing of significant life events or age-related social roles; linked or interdependent lives; and human agency. This perspective constitutes a theoretical lens through which to examine how changes in the conditions, dynamics, and meanings of aging have been brought about by structural and social forces—such as neoliberalism and the spatial reconfiguration of the family—in the context of international migration and transnational care. First, individuals' life courses are affected by the historical eras or worlds in which they live. In the present context of international migration, similarly, the changing political, social, cultural, and economic conditions brought about by neoliberal globalization also impact older people's lives. Global capitalism, facilitated by advances in communication and transportation technologies, has enabled adult migrants' maintenance of much more intimate and enduring relationships with their families—including elderly parents—left behind in home countries than earlier generations (Baldassar, this volume; Baldassar, Baldock, and Wilding 2007; Basch, Schiller, and Blanc 2008). Building on the principles of self-interest, cost-effectiveness, and reduced government spending, the neoliberal state is also characterized by immigration and welfare policies that discriminate against people with little human and financial capital, but promote so-called modern nuclear, wage-earning households that are self-reliant (Leach 2013; Zhou 2013).

Second, Elder (1994) emphasizes, age is imbued with social meanings, such as age-based expectations about the timing of life-course events and roles (e.g., retirement and grandparenthood). In the context of immigration, however, the timing of those things (e.g., caregiving) may be changed or complicated by the geographic separation of families and generations (Clark, Glick, and Bures 2009). When formal childcare resources are not reliable, for instance, informal care provided by grandparents not only represents a culturally *desirable* notion of grandparenthood; more importantly, it suggests that the postponement of these seniors' entry into a post-retirement stage has become *indispensable* to their adult immigrant children's economic survival (Zhou 2012, 2013).

Third, human lives are interdependent, embedded in social relations with kin and significant others across the lifespan. Yet the constant penetration of state borders in migrants' lives has also challenged some taken-for-granted institutions like the family. When a family lives in multiple states—which also means that family members occupy different social positions within different states—family dynamics and generational experiences are also transformed (Levitt and Schiller 2004; Vertovec 2009). Because children's filial responsibility to care for elderly parents is highly valued in Confucian cultures (e.g., China, Korea, and Japan), the emigration of adult children—especially sons—also provokes movement on the part of seniors, so that filial care can still be practiced meaningfully. Yet the changing social, cultural, and economic environment in the host country means that those adult children may not be able or willing to practice filial care themselves; instead, to realize the filial ideal, they may subcontract their filial duties to paid care workers (Lan 2002).

Fourth, given the dynamic features of the life course, individuals use their agency to make decisions and interact with one another. Examples of such agency include seniors' engagement in transnational activities (e.g., transnational care), transnational consciousness (e.g., simultaneous use of the reference frames in two states), adaptation to the changing environment, and identity reconstruction (Levitt and Schiller 2004; Lie 2010; Treas and Mazumdar 2004). Studies of older Korean immigrants in the United States found that they had modest expectations about their children's filial obligations, and their adoption of modified beliefs on filial piety had indeed contributed to positive intergenerational relations in those families (Kauh 1997, 1998). As well, older Indian immigrants in the United States constantly negotiated between the home and host cultures, and developed a sense of being simultaneously here and there that is central to good aging (Lamb 2002). Despite challenges, older immigrants were able to adapt, to various extents, to the changes in their life trajectories resulting from immigration and to create meaning for their lives in a new environment.

Methods

The main purpose of the larger qualitative study (2007–2010), which generated the data presented here, was to understand the dynamics, experiences, and effects of Chinese grandparents' transnational caregiving experiences in Canada. Participants were recruited through multiple social networks, such as Chinese websites and settlement services, and personal referral by research participants in three cities in Ontario, Canada. The data were collected from individual, face-to-face, semistructured, in-depth interviews with thirty-six grandparents (five grandfathers and thirty-one grandmothers) who had come from PRC to care for their grandchildren in Canada. Although the purposive sample of this study may not represent the actual gender distribution of the larger group of Chinese grandparent caregivers, grandmothers are usually primary caregivers, while grandfathers tend to provide both emotional support and some peripheral assistance to the grandmothers, such as by playing with grandchildren, shopping for groceries, and snow shoveling. It is not uncommon for some grandmothers to have come to or stayed in Canada alone to help, either because they were widowed or because their husbands had other commitments (such as care for other family members and higher retirement ages for men) in China.

Written, informed consent was obtained from each participant before the interview. Conducted in Mandarin, the interviews lasted from one and a half to two hours. In addition to the in-depth interviews about participants' experiences of transnational caregiving, some demographic information was collected. Excluding one unknown, these grandparents' ages ranged from fifty-four to seventy-seven, with an average of sixty-four years. Their immigration statuses were divided among "Canadian visitor visa holder" (twenty-seven of thirty-six, including twelve grandparents who had applied for permanent residence), "Canadian permanent resident" (seven of thirty-six), and "(naturalized) Canadian citizen" (two of thirty-six). In terms of housing, nineteen grandparents were living in their children's self-owned houses or apartments as part of a three-generation household, twelve were in shared rental apartments with their children and grandchildren, and five were living alone or in couples in publicly funded seniors' homes.

The audio-taped interviews were transcribed verbatim into Chinese to avoid the loss of nuances within the original narratives; they were translated into English at the stage of results dissemination. After reading through the texts of all transcripts, tentative category labels (such as "international travel," "daily caring activities," "intergenerational relations," and "self-perception") were assigned to the discrete statements of participants. Themes emerged in the process of grouping statements with similar category labels into clusters using an electronic coding system (NVivo) and identifying the relationships among categories. I have been able to use the data analysis to develop the comprehensive synthesis of these themes shown below. To protect participants' identities, pseudonyms are used in this chapter.

A Family in Two Countries: Fragmented Grandparenthood across State Borders

Since welfare restructuring in Canada started in the 1980s, care provision, including childcare, has been either downsized or privatized. The consequences have been heavily borne by socioeconomically disadvantaged groups, such as single mothers, low-income families, and newcomers with limited access to viable financial or social support (Aronson and Neysmith 2006; Man 2002; Michel and Mahon 2002). In China, the erosion of public childcare provision since the economic reforms has meant that grandparents caring for their grandchildren has also become a prerequisite for the participation of young parents, especially women, in the workforce (Cook and Dong 2011; Nyland et al. 2009; Xiao and Cooke 2012). In the context of immigration, the "astronaut family," or the geographically split households, observed among Chinese immigrants in the West (e.g., the United States, Australia, and Canada), is an example of a family-oriented strategy to overcome various socioeconomic challenges in the host country and maximize collective interests; for example, better education or care for the children and better business opportunities or career prospects for the adults (Chee 2005; Chiang 2008; Da 2003; Ong 1999).

The emigration of adult children was commonly viewed by Chinese seniors in this study as a significant change in their lives, given that "a family is now living in two countries." Upon receiving their children's request for child-care, none of the grandparents in this study viewed refusing this request as an option. Caring for grandchildren is a traditional family obligation in Chinese culture, and their children needed their help. Some grandparents even had to leave their own elderly parents or parents-in-law—in their eighties or nineties—behind. Although these relatives had other relatives in China who could provide elder care, as they saw it, their children in Canada had no one else to turn to.

Transnational caregiving was also viewed by seniors as an opportunity for them, as parents and grandparents, to demonstrate the cultural significance of family: "*In China we have a term,* ge dai qing *[intergenerational love]: that is, parents pass their love on to their grandchildren as a way to love their own children. . . . This is a Chinese tradition that I learned from my parents. . . . I want to contribute to our children's and grandchildren's life, and doing so makes me very happy, very proud and satisfied. . . . I think this is what family means*" *(Mr. Li, age sixty years)*. Chinese immigrant families' demand for transnational care does not automatically grant these seniors transnational mobility, however.

To obtain a visitor's visa, older immigrants had to pass a physical checkup and present various kinds of evidence, such as a notarized bank statement and proof of home ownership in China, in order to prove that they had no intention of staying in Canada illegally or beyond the visa's time period. Some seniors had to travel from their hometowns to cities where Canadian embassies or consulates are located, and some of them were rejected the first time, so they had to go back, wait for months, and then reapply. The rejection of their visa applications caused some seniors to miss one of most important and happiest moments of their lives: the birth of the first grandchild. One thrice-rejected older couple missed their daughter's delivery, and their grandchild was already a year old when they finally arrived in Canada. The visa application process was commonly perceived as unnecessarily complicated, restrictive, discriminatory, and expensive. The uncertainty of obtaining a visa told them they were not wanted as grandparents in Canada (e.g., "I felt like Canada does not welcome us as grandparents"), and reinforced their sense of separation from their children. A grandmother commented: "Our children are Canadian citizens now, and our grandchildren are Canadian born. We are their families, but we may not be allowed to go to see them and to care for them when they need us. . . . [The Canadian authorities] don't understand our love for our children; what we care about is not living in Canada, but our children" (Mrs. Gao, age sixty-five). Upon their arrival, as visitors these seniors were usually granted a six-month stay. Most tried to renew their visa for at least another six months in order to avoid disrupting the childcare arrangement. When their visa expired, they had to go back to China; in some cases, they brought their grandchildren with them if no alternative care arrangement could be secured. In this study, twenty-six out of thirty-six grandparents came to Canada more than once (two to four times) for caregiving primarily because of the time restriction on their visitor's visa. In the interviews, some seniors expressed the pain of having to separate, sometimes more than once, from their grandchildren and children. It was not unusual for them to find, to their regret, that the grandchildren they once cared for were, after geographical separation for a couple of years, unable or unwilling to communicate with them in Chinese. They thus also perceived their grandparenthood as fragmented by the time limitations placed on their travel between the two countries. According to them, cultivating a notion of family requires its members to see each other often and to spend time together: "If we are unable to stay together, then family just becomes an abstract term in the end" (Mr. Deng, age sixty-seven). While they were in China, Canada—as the home of their children and grandchildren—continued to be present in their daily lives and thoughts. Ultimately, no matter where these seniors are, they have simultaneously lived at a "home away from home, here and there" (Lamb 2002, 304). These grandparents' lack of control over the time they spend with their children and grandchildren in Canada has also disrupted their kin bonds, their selfhood (parenthood and grandparenthood), and the ideal of aging as a time traditionally linked with certainty, relaxation, and generational reciprocity, and with a sense of connection and satisfaction (Sun 2012).

Many seniors had considered immigration to Canada themselves, primarily because of their desire to travel freely between the two countries, see their grandchildren frequently, and live near their children when they themselves reach the point where they are too old to care for themselves. Of the thirty-six grandparents in the study, seven had become Canadian permanent residents, two had gained Canadian citizenship, and twelve seniors had applied for permanent residence but not yet received it. Although for some immigration was a strategy to obtain greater transnational mobility and proximity to their children, for others it was perceived as the only imperative, because their child in Canada is their only child, or all their children have emigrated from China, as explained by a widowed grandmother:

My son [immigrated to] the USA, and my daughter [immigrated to Canada]. [Like my daughter,] my son and my daughter-in-law also persuaded me to immigrate: "We are unable to care for you when you get even older if you stay in China. It is inconvenient for us to go that far to visit you, even if you can get care at a seniors' home there." My life in China is good; all my friends and siblings are there, and I miss them a lot. I would certainly not apply for immigration [to Canada] if any of my children were in China. So I felt like I didn't have a choice. (Mrs. Dai, age sixty-five)

Proximity to children, associated with their traditional ideal of dependency in old age, is integral to family solidarity and the sense of security and certainty of elderly Asian immigrants in Western contexts (Kauh 1997). In this study, Chinese skilled-immigrant families' need for childcare, exacerbated by both shrinking institutional care provision and pressures of post-immigration survival—including career development—has also facilitated the development of the transnational family. Although paid care workers are mobilized through the global care market with the facilitation of the northern states, the flow of the unpaid kin-based caregivers in my study was primarily driven by cultural notions of family and family obligation, and mediated, if not necessarily inhibited, by Canada's immigration policies. When the care burden has been downloaded to grandparents overseas, however, Canada's implementation of a restrictive and discriminatory border control policy would only increase the socioeconomic risks and inequalities borne by these families. Various constraints (e.g., eligibility and time limit) on Canadian visas have disrupted the process of family construction; they have also further disadvantaged some families with limited resources for financial sponsorship, despite their dire need for care.

International migration, as "a life-long process of complex interaction between individuals and groups who often live far apart" (Lunt 2009, 244), has presented extensive impacts on family: not only for the nuclear families of Chinese skilled immigrants in Canada, but also for their elderly parents living in China or, subsequently, living on a transnational scale between China and Canada. State borders, through such consequences as geographic separation and border crossing, have separated their multigenerational families. This, in turn, has significantly altered the sociocultural conditions in which both immigrant families' childcare arrangements and seniors' transition into old age (including elder care) take place.

Grandparents as Caregivers: Linked Lives across Generations

Upon arrival in Canada, grandparents were immediately integrated into a much faster pace of life. Their typical day started in the early morning with breakfast preparation, and continued until the children and grandchildren went to bed at night. Depending on the children's ages, their childcare workload varied: some completely took over baby care, so that the mothers could go back to work or school, while others primarily took care of grandchildren after day-care hours. Although their children's own contribution to care is expected, this seemed limited for most of the families under study, because most skilled immigrant couples were at the stage of restarting their careers from scratch in Canada and had to be fully committed to their work or study. The older couples usually worked as a team to share care work and housework, while those who came alone often reported physical burnout. Because their son-in-law was working in another city and their daughter was getting her doctorate, for example, one older couple had become the primary caregivers for their three-month-old grandchild. The grandmother described their daily life as follows:

> My main task is to care for the baby, and my husband is in charge of cooking and grocery shopping. My daughter just finished writing her dissertation, but she is still very busy, because now she has started job hunting. So childcare is basically my job, except that my daughter has to breastfeed the baby. . . . She has not had a good night's sleep because of breastfeeding. So I take the baby away from her room around 6 a.m. every day, so that she can sleep for a while. . . . If she were taking care of the baby on her own, I don't think she could even find time to eat. (Mrs. Wang, age fifty-five)

Viewing their time with their grandchildren as rewarding and happy, seniors also made such comments as, "My life here is physically tiresome but spiritually fulfilled" (Mrs. Ruan, age sixty-one) and "I feel like I am aging more slowly when I stay with my grandchild" (Mrs. Fang, age sixty-nine).

Seniors' appreciation of their children's struggles in this new country meant that they also viewed their uncompensated transnational care as a way to support their children in their efforts to catch up with native Canadians. According to them, if they did those "meaningless" household chores, their immigrant children could spend that time on their career development or with their own children; and if they could help their immigrant families save money through unpaid childcare, their children could have more resources for other things, like further education and house buying. Since their adult immigrant children usually did not have the time required for their own children's development, some grandparents saw themselves as surrogates, normalizing their grandchildren's childhood and growth. Feeling her body "being overdrawn by five years" (aging accelerated by a heavy workload), one grandmother nonetheless tried to renew her visa a couple more times: "If I can work hard for one more day, that means the life of my daughter's family can be smooth for another day" (Mrs. Chen, age unknown). The sentiment was echoed by another grandmother: "Why do we have to work so hard here? . . . My understanding is that my daughter could work less if I worked more. . . . I want her to live a better life, right? So if I take good care of these two grandchildren, then my daughter will have peace of mind and can concentrate on her work. And then they will have a better life in the future" (Mrs. Wen, age sixty-three). These seniors' experiences in Canada and on a transnational scale echo the principle of "linked or interdependent lives" in life-course theory (Elder 1994, 5); that is, adult immigrant children's settlement process in Canada has postponed their elderly parents' entry into a post-retirement stage and, thus, also prolonged their active and substantial contributions to the lives of the former's families.

Coining the term "family time economy," Jane M. Maher, Jo Lindsay, and Suzanne Franzway (2008) argue that women's time for work depends on the time required for caregiving and family, given that one's time is limited and time for care (especially for dependents) is less flexible. In this light, it is important to recognize the multiple links between Chinese grandparents' unpaid caregiving and immigrants' family economy and welfare. The politics and policies of care that have devalued and ignored such nonmonetary care resources as time (not only time for unpaid care, but also time with family), emotion, and cultural knowledge, which are key to children's development and overall family well-being, must be critically reappraised. Maliha Safri and Julie Graham (2010) argue that a global household, consisting of immigrants and their families left behind, is an everyday site for both capitalist and noncapitalist production (e.g., care, affection, and social wealth). Its noncapitalist production has significant aggregate economic values, in part because of the economic and emotional interdependence of household members despite their geographic dispersion. Although the dominant institutional approaches to social redistribution is through taxation and welfare systems and to care redistribution through global care chains, Chinese transnational families, indeed, have exerted a similar redistributive influence through mobilizing and allocating various care resources across generations and countries: in particular, from the older generation to the younger generations, and from China to Canada.

The "Three Nots" Identity: Changing Intergenerational Relations in the New Country

The arrival of grandparents also transformed immigrants' nuclear families into three-generation households for nineteen of the thirty-six participants in the study. Some were happy about the new living arrangements; others, however, found that they had to cope with challenges such as crowded living conditions, conflicts with in-laws, and communication problems resulting from cultural and generational gaps. During interviews, grandparents also talked about a few cases when seniors had to end their caregiving and return to China because of difficulties coping with the constrained living space and intergenerational conflicts. Some seniors tried to assume the role of traditional parental authority but often encountered resistance. After witnessing the negative effects of her interference in her daughter's career and conjugal relationship, for instance, a sixty-five-year-old grandmother finally realized that she had to "learn how to be an elder" in Canada. "As an elder I should not have dominated or interfered in my daughter's life." She commented: "I should accept my [secondary] place in my daughter's home, and that my advice does not work here [in Canada]" (Mrs. Qian, age sixty-five). After being baptized in Canada, two seniors also attributed their positive intergenerational relationships to their willingness to surrender their Chinese traditional parental authority, following the Bible's assertions about the (nuclear) family and the men's—that is to say, their sons-in-law's—roles as heads of their houses.

Many also felt neglected or alienated by insufficient communication with their adult children. This, combined with their limited interactions with the outside world, exacerbated these seniors' sense of isolation. Some joked about their awkward "three nots identity," a coined term widely circulated among older Chinese caregivers in their children's homes: not a master (because they cannot make decisions for the families), not a guest (because they have to do care work and housework), and not a servant (because they are not paid), as the following remarks illustrate:

I feel like I came here just to help them, and this is not my home. (Mrs. Zhen, age sixty-four)

[My child's family] are nice to me, but I feel like a subordinate in their lives. (Mrs. Sun, age seventy-three)

I feel like an outsider in Canada. My children are Canadians now, and I am just a guest visiting them. (Mrs. Gao)

The language barrier was the first and foremost difficulty when grandparents interacted outside their children's homes. Although some seniors tried to learn English when their childcare burden lightened as their grandchildren got older, their lack of English proficiency greatly constrained their ability to accomplish small tasks like shopping, conversing, and seeing a doctor, which in turn led to their frustration, feelings of dependence on their children, and low self-esteem, as explained by two grandmothers:

One day my grandchild had a high fever, and his parents were not around. My husband and I were unable to take her to see a doctor because we cannot speak English. So we had to call her father to come back to take her to the doctor. If we had been in China, I would have taken her myself right away. But we are able to do very little here. (Mrs. Zhao, age sixty)

In China I at least felt like an intellectual, an educated woman. But here I am just a stay-at-home caregiver; I feel illiterate, deaf-mute and blind [because of language barriers]! I cannot do things without the help of my daughter or son-in-law. . . . So now I have this low self-esteem. . . . I accept that now I am old and out of date. I accept that this is who I am now. (Mrs. Qian)

Living a transnational life has helped Chinese seniors acquire various kinds of knowledge that were not available to them in China, such as knowledge of international travel, English, driving, Western notions of parenthood and the nuclear family, and even, a new religion. Meanwhile, seniors' new lives in Canada have challenged and destabilized their aging identities, which have become increasingly unstable, fluid, and contested as parents, grandparents, caregivers, and visitors or residents in Canada. Yet their changing self-identifications are not only a reflection of a postmodern world (Estes, Biggs, and Philipson 2010), but also an illustration of contradictory sociocultural and structural forces in the context of transnational caregiving. When those seniors' time is integrated into their immigrant children's economic survival and family well-being as an unreciprocated sacrifice, aging has also become a process subordinated to the changing life priorities of their immigrant children's families and to the neoliberal economy.

The timing of seniors' immigration in their life course also makes it more difficult to adapt to the new environment in view of the lifelong connections and familiarity with the home country and culture (Treas 2008). Unlike their skilled immigrant children, whose integration in Canada as the adopted country is key to their future lives, these seniors' relationship with Canada is primarily mediated by their relationships with their children and grandchildren. Their constrained ability to interact with the host society also means that their adult children's families or households have become a key, if not the sole, site in which they organize their everyday lives and negotiate their aging identities; their relationships with their children's families thus remain significant for their sense of well-being in Canada. For those immigrant seniors, the homeland remains a more important reference system (e.g., in such forms as cultural preference, memory, nostalgia, and personal aspirations) than Canada for their daily decisions, sense making, and identity reconstruction. Their adaptation to the new environment is more about accepting various changes in their own and their children's lives than about their own assimilation in Canada. Despite these seniors' agency in self-transformation, it is also important to note, on one hand, how their capacities for and ways of participating in transnational social spaces differ from those of their adult children and, on the other, how interactions with state institutions affect older adults' differential power in transnational families (Basch, Schiller, and Blanc 2008).

Compromised Filial Piety: The Ruptured Generational Reciprocity

The Chinese traditional norm of filial piety (*xiao*) emphasizes children's duty to care for their parents when they age (Hwang 2008; Lai and Leonenko 2007). Citing a Chinese phrase *shang ci xia xiao* (loving parents and then filial children), seniors often see filial piety not as simply children's responsibility to love and care for their elderly parents, but as one aspect of generational reciprocity in everyday family life. Many attributed the continued cultivation of filial piety to traditional multigenerational households: for example, "Three of my four children were brought up by their grandmother, so [they] have learned well to respect them since they were very young" (Mrs. Sun); and, "My daughter grew up by watching how I cared for my own mother every day" (Mrs. Chen). Yet the emigration of adult children in China has not only changed the family structure through which resources and cultural values are transmitted across generations; it has also shaken the family-based welfare system in which elder care is provided (Zhou 2012).

Changing intergenerational relationships and what they perceived as the temporary nature of the three-generation household also affected these seniors' expectations about their immigrant children's ability to fulfill the duties of filial piety. After referring to their own devoted filial care for their elderly parents, many said that they would not expect their immigrant children to do the same for them, given their children's long-term struggles and the different norms of elder care in Canada. Instead, they tended to give more attention to the *ideal* of filial piety or its spiritual aspects, such as love, care, and happiness, than to its practical and material aspects, such as coresidence, day-to-day care, and financial support. Asked about their understanding of filial piety in the context of immigration, some simply defined it in such terms as, "They care about me" (Mrs. Sun), "I am in their hearts" (Mr. Deng, age sixty-seven), or "They respect me" (Mrs. Gu, age sixty-nine); others emphasized their children's filial duty in terms of inculcating traditional notions of the family and Chinese identity in their grandchildren's generation, but were not sure they would do so. For instance, they wished that their children would teach their grandchildren that "grandparents are part of the family" (Mrs. Fang), and that their grandchildren would remember their Chinese heritage and be able to speak Chinese in order to communicate with the greater family in China in the future.

Those who were explicit about not considering immigration often had better living conditions in China, and worried that their immigration would further compromise their children's quality of life in Canada. Although Canada was commonly praised as having an excellent natural environment, a well-developed health-care system, and generally better living conditions, many also perceived that they could live a much more independent and autonomous life in China because of their ability to access their pension, housing, social support, and so on. Although their pension was worth little in Canada after it was exchanged into Canadian dollars, it was enough for them to hire a stay-at-home caregiver in China. If they decided to stay in China, however, they might end up aging alone. This issue may become even more salient, given that Chinese immigrants of the one-child-policy generation (those born in the 1980s and later) have arrived in Canada; the effects of their immigration on elder care should be observed, because two married adult immigrants will have to support and care for four seniors (parents and parents-in-law). Although grandparents appeared to accept the one-way nature of their contribution to and sacrifice for their children's and grandchildren's lives, a helpless and hopeless tone also permeated their narratives in the interviews: for example, "Even if my daughter [in Canada] is filial enough to quit her job to care for me, how can they live without income?" (Mrs. Wang).

Although elderly immigration means that they are no longer separated from their children and grandchildren, aging in a foreign country also makes these seniors more vulnerable to social and health risks like poverty and social isolation (Lai 2004; Lai and Leonenko 2007). The seniors who had successfully immigrated to Canada nevertheless had to cope with various practical challenges, including problems of income security, housing, and separation, again because of their children's relocation in or outside Canada. Many remain financially dependent on their immigrant children, primarily because they needed at least ten years' residence to be eligible for Old Age Security (OAS), a minimum income assistance program in Canada. Although living with children often complicated the relationships of the nuclear families, living alone also meant an extra financial burden for their immigrant children who subsidized the former's living costs. Currently living in a publicly funded seniors' home, for instance, a sixty-nine-year-old widowed grandmother still had to wait three years before she was eligible for OAS, and her only income was 300 Canadian dollars per month from her only child, whose employment had been unstable since coming to Canada. A devoted Christian now, she has accepted her situation, and become a volunteer for Mandarin-speaking counseling in her church. Living on 600 Canadian dollars per month given by her son, similarly, a seventy-seven-year-old grandmother and her husband have been in a seniors' home since her son's family had moved to the United States for employment. They were left behind in part because of the health-care coverage and social welfare programs available to them as Canadian permanent residents. At the time of the interview, her husband had just broken his leg and was unable to move for weeks. Perceiving the care work as too heavy for her at this age, she felt they had now reached the point of seriously considering going back to China, where their daughter was living:

> In the past couple of years we have clearly felt we are aging; both memory and energy are deteriorating. . . . All of a sudden I easily get tired, and always want to take a break. . . . Now that my husband has fallen and broken his leg, and my whole body feels sore all the time, I am thinking perhaps it's time for us to go back. . . . People know when they reach that point, when they feel unable to take care of themselves any more. (Mrs. Wu, age seventy-seven)

Seeing that "Canada is a paradise for children, but not for the elderly" (Mrs. Chen), some immigrant seniors saw China as the place to receive elder care. They often quoted a cultural phrase—*luo ye gui geng* (fallen leaves of a tree finally go to their root)—to indicate their preference to die or to be buried in the homeland. Regardless of their immigrant status and the country where they end up living, the transnational ties between China and Canada have become integral to their later lives.

The emigration of adult children has also interrupted the functioning of the family as an important mechanism of exchanging resources across generations in Chinese culture, where the extended family plays an essential role in welfare and care provision for the elderly (Wu and Hart 2002; Zhan and Montgomery 2003). Although seniors' transnational care and later immigration were driven by the traditional notion of family, such a notion has become increasingly selective for adult children, and even abstract for the grandchildren's generation. The disrupted character of transnational households and the difficult settlement of immigrant families also made it challenging to carry on Chinese traditions that emphasize reciprocal responsibilities across generations. The processes of modernization and immigration have eroded some aspects of filial piety, such as cash payment from adult children to elderly parents, multigenerational cohabitation, and filial care, in Chinese cities and among overseas Chinese immigrants (Cheung and Kwan 2009; Lan 2002; Liber, Nihira, and Mink 2004). Although some seniors were able, to some degree, to adopt the modified tradition, the *practical* aspects of filial piety as an elder-care model are still crucial for those with limited access to resources, whether private or public (Chou 2011; Sung and Kim 2002). Despite these changes, as illustrated by this study, the *ideal* of filial piety remains important for both the grandparent and the child generations because it is so tightly associated with cultural identity and the seniors' quality of life.

From the perspective of social welfare, furthermore, such a cultural rupture suggests not only the exploitative, one-way intergenerational redistribution of informal resources (emotion and unpaid care), but also the gap between immigrants' needs for care in relation to changing family structures and the delayed government policy response to such changes. The increasing interconnections between elderly parents' and their immigrant children's lives suggest new insights into the life course that is usually considered on an individual basis in a domestic context. That is, the later lives of the Chinese seniors under study are not simply, or at least not entirely, linear or causal results of their own experiences in their earlier life stages in China, but are also determined by the immigration experiences of their children's families in Canada, and of their subsequent multistranded connections with both China and Canada.

Conclusion

Critical gerontologists see aging as a social construction that includes the intersections of microprocesses with the macrolevel forces of individual aging experiences (Elder 1994; Estes, Biggs, and Phillipson 2010). In the contexts of international migration and transnationalism, however, both the macrostructural conditions and microindividual experiences of aging have become further diversified and complicated. I argue that the life trajectories of Chinese grandparents in this study have been transformed by their adult children's immigration to Canada and subsequent settlement challenges into transnational processes that are *simultaneously* shaped by various individual, familial, cultural, and structural contexts in both Canada and China. Meanwhile, various forms of cross-country connections, such as the material, cognitive, emotional, and symbolic, resulting from transnational care and/or elderly migration have permeated the everyday lives of these seniors and, in turn, changed their experiences of aging and the meanings they attribute to it. The emigration of these seniors' adult children has transformed the seniors' aging trajectories from a traditional life stage "in place" into a complex transnational process. However, the close intersections of these seniors' lives with those of their adult immigrant children also suggest the continued relevance of kin-based generational relationships to these grandparents' later lives.

The critical examination of aging in the context of transnational care helps us take into consideration those dimensions—such as changing family structure, transnational mobility, cultural rupture, informal care resource redistribution across generations and countries, and policy effects going beyond state borders and the nuclear family—that are changed by immigration and globalization.

It allows us to rethink aging from a perspective broader than the individual that links seniors' experiences with their relationships with other family members and interactions with macrostructures. The findings of this study also affirm the relevance of intergenerational family relationships, geography, and migrant status in the contexts of international migration and transnationalism to the reconfiguration of power dynamics and inequalities in individuals' later lives, in addition to other more commonly identified factors, such as gender, class, ethnicity, and "race." The various inequalities that pervade the new life trajectories of Chinese seniors in a transnational context also reveal the contradictory nature of globalization's social, economic, cultural, and political processes, and the importance of developing knowledge about transnational aging in order to inform effective practices, policies, and substantial structural changes at local, national, and transnational levels.

The challenging relationships among care, aging, immigration, and social policy presented in this chapter also call for rethinking the relationships of the national with the transnational, given that globalization means "not the dissolution of the nation-state, but the unsettling presence of the 'world' within the nation-state" (Clarke 2005, 409). To reduce the generational and transnational inequalities perpetuated in the caregiving experiences under discussion, for instance, states, especially the receiving countries in the north, should lower barriers to entry of unpaid kin-based caregivers and recognize the care interdependencies across generations, countries, and sectors in this globalizing and interconnected world. Domestic social policy makers and analysts should be aware of, and take into account, the policy effects that go beyond the nation-state and its citizenry, and intersect with other aspects of immigration, such as the spatial reconfiguration of the family, cultural change, and aging. Without timely policy responses to such transnational welfare connections or interdependence across generations, countries, and different policy areas, there are some long-term consequences to be borne by these grandparents, as well as by their families.

ACKNOWLEDGMENTS

I wish to express my appreciation to Chinese seniors who participated in this study and to Liping Peng, Xiaoxin Ji, Xieqing Lin, Winnie Lo, Mingwei Zhang, Huijing Yang, and Natasha Vattikonda for their assistance at the different stages of this research project. This work was carried out with the aid of the Social Sciences and Humanities Research Council of Canada (SSHRCC) Standard Research Grant (2007–2010).

3

Sacrifice or Abandonment?

Nicaraguan Grandmothers' Narratives of Migration as Kin Work

KRISTIN ELIZABETH YARRIS

Norma and Angela are vibrant Nicaraguan women in their fifties whose lives have been transformed by transnational migration across time even though they themselves have not emigrated. Living on opposite sides of Managua, the capital city of Nicaragua, Norma and Angela do not know each other, and yet their family circumstances have many parallels: both women's husbands emigrated to the United States decades earlier; both are mothers of daughters who migrated ten years ago; and both are primary caregivers for young grandchildren, the children of these migrant mothers. As intergenerational caregivers in transnational families, Angela and Norma have been pushed to respond to migration and its effects on their family lives; first, as wives, then, as mothers, now, as grandmothers. As caregivers in the present, these women form strong emotional ties to their grandchildren, accomplishing the kin work of raising children and managing households in Nicaragua, while simultaneously fostering ties of relationality in transnational families divided by space and time.

Despite the similarities in the circumstances surrounding migration, Angela and Norma have responded differently to the prospect of their grandchildren's reunification with migrant mothers abroad. For her part, Angela is filled with ambivalence at the prospect of granddaughter Laleska's migration, worrying about the girl's increasingly troubled relationship with her mother (Angela's daughter) Karla, concerned that the young girl will have difficulty adjusting to her new family in Miami, and even more apprehensive about the emptiness she herself will feel when Laleska leaves. For Angela, migration represents a threat to the unity and togetherness she values in her family. Of Karla's migration, Angela says, "It's not the same having her face-to-face, being able to be with her in person as talking to her over the telephone." These tensions in transnational mother-child ties consume Angela's caregiving, as she struggles against the looming possibility that migration may ultimately result in abandonment of family members in Nicaragua.

Norma, on the other hand, has oriented her care for her grandson Jeremy much more unequivocally around her sense that migration is a necessary sacrifice made for family members. Thus, Norma and Jeremy look forward to his future reunification with mother María José with anticipation. Norma has reinforced the idea that Jeremy will leave to join his mother abroad ever since María José left more than ten years ago, orienting her caregiving with this plan in mind. Of the unknown future surrounding Jeremy's departure, Norma says, "I'm not fearful, what I feel is desire to see mother and son reunited." For Norma, Jeremy's reunification with Mariá José in the United States represents the culmination of a decade of her kin work, carefully oriented toward sustaining the relationship between mother and son across borders within the frame of migration as sacrifice.

In this chapter, I argue that understanding transnational migration and its consequences for kinship and care requires an intergenerational perspective, one that attends to the ways caregivers utilize narratives to render significance from the disruptions and disjunctures of migration over time. Grandmothers who assume care for grandchildren in response to mothers' migration bring to intergenerational caregiving and to transnational kin work their personal experiences of living with migration in the past. More specifically, women's experiences of their husbands' migrations decades earlier open the possibilities of two competing narrative frames—migration as sacrifice and migration as abandonment—with which women engage to make sense of their daughters' migrations in the present and of the uncertain prospect of their grandchildren's migrations in the future. Grandmothers weave narratives to make meaning of the tensions, troubles, and uncertainties of transnational family life, and thus give significance to migration over time and across generations. However, although grandmothers work to sustain a narrative of migration as a sacrifice made for family well-being, the counter narrative of migration as abandonment constantly threatens to undo the narrative of sacrifice. In the face of these threats, narratives of migration are a form of care, utilized by grandmother caregivers over time to uphold values for unity and relationality in transnational families.

An Intergenerational Perspective on Migration

Grandmother caregiving is an essential resource for families divided by national borders, even though women of the *tercera edad*, or third age, have been largely overlooked in studies of transnational families (Abrego 2014; Dreby 2010) and global care chains (Parreñas 2001, 2005; Yeates 2005). Grandmother caregivers draw on past experiences of migration in responding to the present realities of their daughters' migrations and, in turn, to their grandchildren's experiences of their mother's migration. Rather than viewing responses to present-day migration as overdetermined by the past, I maintain that understanding contemporary migration experiences requires situating them within family histories, shared memories, and lingering emotional responses from prior generations. Specifically, an intergenerational perspective considers how past migrations shape grandmothers' responses to contemporary migration, and in turn, how past and present weave together to influence how families perceive the possibility of future migrations.

Applying an intergenerational perspective toward care work and kin work in transnational families moves the frame outward—across time and generations, and into extended kin relations. As Cati Coe (2016) has recently argued, migration reconfigures time and temporality as well as distance and spatiality. In particular, transnational families must reorder cultural expectations for care across the life course in response to the temporal disjunctures wrought by migration. Here, I follow Coe in making temporality central to my analysis of transnational family life, considering time in terms of generations and life course, such that an individual or a family experiences contemporary migration in light of what has transpired in the past and what is anticipated (or feared) for the future. In doing so, I show that caregivers' and children's understandings of migration are shaped by broader relational dynamics and family histories, enacted through relations of care proffered by surrogate caregivers (in this case, grandmothers).

In developing my intergenerational perspective on care in transnational families, I build upon both a life-course perspective as well as recent anthropological thinking about age and globalization. A life-course approach highlights three temporal dimensions: individual time, family time, and historical time (Hareven 1994, 439). Within public health, a life-course perspective is applied to reveal the cumulative health impacts on an individual across the course of an individual life. This perspective is important in broadening the analytic frame to consider not just contemporary risks to health or threats to well-being, but how individual responses to contemporary threats are informed by previous life experiences, particularly experiences of hardship.[1] In anthropology, Jennifer Cole and Deborah Durham have argued that understanding experiences of age and aging within contemporary globalization benefits from a perspective that foregrounds both time and generation. Cole and Durham use the concept of "regeneration" to refer to the "mutually constitutive interplay between intergenerational relations and wider historical and social processes" (2007, 17). Whereas attention to social reproduction highlights the ways gender and kinship intersect through roles and responsibilities to shape household care-giving labor, this concept implies a static *reproduction* of social and cultural life, leaving little room for flexibility, negotiation, or change. On the other hand, as Cole and Durham suggest, the term "regeneration" captures a processual sense of culture changing over time and across generations. An intergenerational perspective can thus capture both the cumulative impacts of social experience on an individual life, as well as the ways individuals respond to the social and cultural changes associated with migration by reconfiguring relations of care and kinship.

In addition to attending to cumulative individual life events and the regeneration of social and cultural life over time, an intergenerational perspective also captures a sense of generation in socialhistorical time. That is, a generational perspective must consider individuals in time, as they share a social experience of historical events and their cultural consequences (Mannheim [1952] 1972). As individuals and groups, people carry the experience of belonging to a historical cohort throughout their lives, and this experience shapes their response to social and cultural changes over time (see also Cole 2007). In this analysis of Nicaraguan transnational families, I show how women's experiences of migration at a specific sociohistorical moment following the 1979 Sandinista Revolution reverberate over time, and their narrations contour their responses to migration in subsequent generations. More concretely, women tend to frame their husbands' migrations in the 1980s as necessary responses to the political and economic insecurity of the Contra War and the concomitant US economic embargo against Nicaragua. Given these powerful historical events, migration was viewed as a move made to provide for the well-being of families, and an extension of gendered cultural expectations that fathers should provide economic security for their children. However, this initial framing of migration did not hold up over time, as some male migrants failed to live up to expectations that as fathers they would provide economic and instrumental support to their children. In response, a counter-narrative emerged in this first generation, where women (as wives) situated migration as their husbands' ultimate abandonment of family members back home.

In a second generation, women experience their daughters' decisions to emigrate against the historical backdrop of economic scarcity and inequality that characterize the neoliberal and post-neoliberal periods in Nicaragua, where migration is largely a response to material hardship, poverty, and un- and under-employment (Rocha 2006). In this generation, women (as mothers) respond to their daughters' migrations by again drawing on the frame of sacrifice to make sense of migration as a necessary move made by mothers to provide for their children, even as they must renegotiate gendered expectations for care as a result, with mothers sacrificing through work abroad and grandmothers sharing in the sacrifice of migration by assuming care of grandchildren in Nicaragua.

In the third generation, children face an uncertain future where the possibility of their reunification with migrant mothers abroad is determined by geopolitical forces and immigration policies beyond their control. Here, the realities of families of migrants are shaped by increasingly restrictive immigration policies, which delimit mother migrants' abilities to obtain legal residency for themselves and their children. In response, children and their caregivers are left dealing with the uncertainty surrounding children's potential reunification with mothers abroad. Women (as grandmothers) respond to these uncertainties by crafting narratives that counter disconnection and foster relationality across generations and borders. Narratives are thus a central part of transnational kin work, helping caregivers and other family members make the disjunctures of migration significant given both broad historical transformations and local cultural expectations of family sacrifice and care.

Narratives and Grandmothers' Transnational Kin Work

In this chapter, I consider narrative both as an ethnographic object, that is, a form of care that sustains the meaning of migration for those experiencing it, and as an analytical approach, that is, a way of interpreting the cultural significance of the stories told about migration. In engaging with a narrative approach to migration and care, I am informed by the ways medical anthropologists have used narrative theory to uncover the significance that health and illness have for individuals in relation to culturally valued life courses (Garro and Mattingly 2000; Mattingly 2014). Such an approach links individual experience to broader cultural meanings and calls attention to the role of narrator and audience in the cocreation of narratives (Garro and Mattingly 2000, 25). In this examination of Nicaraguan transnational families, two narrative frames emerge from and respond to family members' experiences of migration over the generations: migration as sacrifice and migration as abandonment. These narratives are stitched together tenuously, one always existing alongside the possibility of the other. In this way, narratives are generative and practical; they help grandmother caregivers and other family members make meaning out of migration. This meaning is shared and negotiated within families as they confront the challenges of transnational life and attempt to regenerate cultural values for unity in family relationships over time and across borders.

Grandmother caregivers in transnational families are responsible not just for everyday social reproduction, essential as that is to the health and wellbeing of their children and families, but also for the regeneration of family life over time and across borders. Michaela di Leonardo conceived of women's roles in maintaining emotional connection within families as part of their "kinwork," which includes activities necessary to maintain "a sense of family," whether organizing family reunions, coordinating holiday celebrations, or sending written letters (di Leonardo 1987, 443). Loretta Baldassar has extended the concept of kin work to describe women's work within transnational families, including the emotional labor needed to maintain ties between migrant mothers and the (grand)children in their care across time, distance, and national borders (2007, 387). In their roles as primary caregivers, grandmothers engage in the daily activities of kin work for the children in their care: feeding, bathing, clothing, and supervising schooling; grandmothers also mediate the emotional relations between children and mothers living abroad. As such, grandmothers engage in the three dimensions of caring labor outlined by Evelyn Nakano Glenn (2010, 5): direct care of persons, household maintenance, and fostering social relationships. Grandmothers' kin work is accomplished as women enter later life facing the reality that migration has upended cultural expectations for care across generations in such a way that, instead of their adult daughters caring for them, grandmothers now care for grandchildren. Although this situation represents cultural disruption, women also find pleasure and meaning in grandmothering, drawing on past experiences of mothering.[2]

The creation of narrative frames that render the disruptions of transnational migration meaningful is a central dimension of grandmother care and kin work. Grandmothers craft narratives over time, through the prism of emotionally charged experiences of their husbands' migrations in the past, and through interactions with their migrant daughters and grandchildren in the present. Grandmothers tell stories of migration, signal key family events, and encourage appropriate actions and reactions from family members. As primary caregivers, grandmothers assume responsibility for socializing children's emotions, shaping their responses to mother migration, and mediating their relationships to migrant mothers over the distance and time that characterize transnational family life. Over time, migration is alternately cast as a necessary sacrifice for the sake of children and families, or as a form of abandonment of family members; the ability to sustain the narrative of migration as sacrifice depends on social and historical circumstances and on individual and interpersonal responses to migration. Further, narratives are relational and processual, shared within families across generations, as a way of regenerating family and cultural values in the face of disjunctures and tensions. For instance, children participate in family narratives, adopting or contesting the narrative frames given to mother migration and asserting significance based on their experiences (Rae-Espinoza 2011). Grandmothers engage with these contestations, crafting the meaning of migration for themselves and the children in their care in ways that respond to present tensions and future uncertainties while drawing on past experiences.

Overview of the Research

This chapter draws on ethnographic research I conducted with twenty-four Nicaraguan transnational families in Managua, Nicaragua, and surrounding communities over eleven months of fieldwork from 2009 to 2010 and on three subsequent shorter visits. Elsewhere, I have described the procedures and methods of this research in detail (Yarris 2014b). Here, I present the cases of two families from this research study. Both are headed by women (Angela and Norma) who are grandmothers—primary caretakers of the children of mother migrants.[3] In both families, as with all families in my study, I conducted a series of semistructured interviews and engaged in hours of informal conversations and everyday activities with grandmothers, children, and other coresident family members. I interviewed Norma's migrant daughter, María José, on the occasion of her return visit to Nicaragua and I have spoken with Angela's daughter, Karla, by phone several times. I remain in contact with both families through phone calls, Facebook, and WhatsApp messaging.

Two Transnational Families

I have selected to present Angela and Norma's families in this analysis of narratives and transnational care in large part because the two women share much in common, and yet orient differently toward the promises and perils of migration. Through these similarities and differences, we can see how grandmothers draw on narratives as part of their kin work in an effort to contend with the troubles and uncertainties of transnational family life.

Both Angela and Norma experienced the outmigration of their husbands to the United States, both men leaving their wives in Nicaragua to care for children with the promise that migration would result in better futures for their families.[4] Although the circumstances surrounding these migrations differ, both men ultimately lost contact with their Nicaraguan spouses and children, a loss that reverberates through Angela and Norma's narratives of migration. In a second generation of migration, Angela and Norma are both primary caretakers for grandchildren whose mothers emigrated when they were approximately one year old. These children, Norma's grandson Jeremy and Angela's granddaughter Laleska, were each eleven years old at the time of this research, meaning Norma and Angela have been raising their respective grandchild for over ten years. Norma's daughter María José and Angela's daughter Karla both emigrated to the United States and experienced difficulties associated with a lack of legal documentation, instability, and insecurity during the first years of life in the United States. Each woman has since married, gained legal residency, and had US-born children. Neither Jeremy nor Laleska have met their half siblings in person. However, both children in Nicaragua live in households shared with extended family; in addition to their grandmothers, Jeremy and Laleska live in proximity to cousins, uncles, and aunts who are also involved to a limited extent in their care.

Further, both migrant mothers have consistently communicated and sent remittances since settling in the United States. Angela and Norma manage the money their daughters send home and allocate it toward children's care; namely, schooling, food, clothing, and medical costs.[5] In each case, there is a prospect of the child's reunification with the mother in the United States, since Karla and María José have been processing the legal paperwork necessary for family reunification visas. However, Angela and Norma encounter the possibility of their grandchild's reunification differently: Angela is ambivalent; Norma is unequivocally supportive. It is in this difference that the role of narratives as a central part of intergenerational caregiving in transnational families becomes most clear. Norma is able to uphold the narrative of migration as sacrifice to frame her daughter's migration to her grandson; however, a counter-narrative of migration as abandonment influences Angela's interpretation of migration within her family, impacting granddaughter Laleska's orientation toward migration in a third generation. In the analysis that follows, I trace Angela and Norma's experiences with migration across three generations in order to show how narratives are construed over time, such that past experiences shape how women respond to mother migration in the present, and how the past and present influence how grandmothers and grandchildren respond to the uncertain prospect of children's future reunification with mothers abroad.

The First Generation: Migration as Abandonment

For Norma and Angela, the migration of their husbands in an earlier generation held the promise of worthwhile sacrifice but ultimately ended in abandonment. Although the circumstances of these men's migrations differ, both left Nicaragua for the United States promising greater security and stability for their wives and families. Norma and Angela initially supported their husbands' decisions to emigrate because of their belief that migration would improve their families' circumstances; however, within a few years of their departure, each woman began to experience her husband's migration as a form of abandonment. First, both men failed to send regular monetary remittances back to Nicaragua, shattering the illusion that migration would improve family economic circumstances. Second, and perhaps the source of even greater disillusionment, their adult children (Norma's daughters Vanesa and María José and Angela's children Karla and Jonathan) left Nicaragua in order to reunite with their fathers in Miami, even though their fathers had failed to support them in the past. This failure was exacerbated by the fact that the men had formed new families in the United States, information relayed back to Norma and Angela by their migrant children, and heightening the women's sense of abandonment. For both, their prior experience with migration colors their responses to their daughters' migrations decades later and shapes how they respond to the prospect of their grandchildren's future reunification with mothers in the current generation.

Norma's husband, Manlo, left Nicaragua for the United States in the mid-1980s for reasons Norma describes as "*persecución política*" (political persecution). Manlo had served as an officer in the infamous army of Nicaragua's former US-backed dictator Anastasio Somoza. After the Sandinista Revolution in 1979, in which the popular Frente Sandinista de Liberación Nacional (Sandinista Front of National Liberation, or FSLN) ousted Somoza, members of the regime's Guardia Nacional (National Guard) were disbanded. Former soldiers like Manlo were stigmatized in the new revolutionary society, associated with the atrocities and human rights violations of the Somoza regime, and viewed by many Sandinistas as traitors, "Liberals," who had aligned with the dictator and, by extension, US imperialism.[6] For Manlo, such stigma closed the doors to employment possibilities; for Norma and the rest of the family, it resulted in feeling ostracized from their neighbors, who pointed to Manlo's past as the reason he and his family should suffer hardship. Norma remembers that her neighbors questioned whether she and her family deserved the house they lived in: "They said this was a Somoza house, that I was a Liberal and for that reason the [Somoza] regime had given me this house." Given this hostile climate, when Manlo told Norma he was leaving for the United States, she viewed his departure as necessary to salvage the reputation and well-being of her family. Manlo fled to Miami, leaving Norma as a single mother caring for her four young children, aged three to ten years at the time.[7]

Norma retains anti-Sandinista sentiments shaped by her family's history. For instance, because Norma struggled to feed her children after her husband left, she blames the FSLN for the food shortages that plagued the country in the 1980s. Norma remembers, "There wasn't enough to eat; there wasn't enough to drink; there weren't enough shoes." Norma recalled how these insecurities pushed her and other single mothers to cross by river into Honduras to obtain milk for their children. Norma narrates this period as a story of necessary sacrifice of fathers and mothers; while her husband was pushed out of Nicaragua by political forces, she and thousands of other women crossed national borders in search of food for their children.[8] Norma continues to hold the FSLN responsible for pushing Nicaraguans like her husband and her daughters to emigrate to seek political and economic security. This view is central to her narrative of migration as a necessary sacrifice.

Although Norma initially viewed her husband's migration as indispensable to their family's well-being, this view was challenged by the realities of transnational life as they played out over time. In fact, Manlo never sent remittances despite his promises to do so, leading Norma to feel "he forgot that his children existed." Within a few years of his departure, Norma found out through relatives and transborder rumor networks that Manlo had settled with a (Nicaraguan) wife in Miami with whom he had two children. This knowledge cemented her realization that her husband would no longer support his family in Nicaragua. Norma's response was to overcome her feelings of disillusionment and commit to raising her children to the best of her abilities, in part to prove to Manlo that she could be a successful mother without him. She recalled feeling, "I'm going to show him that I can be mother and father" and repeating to herself, "I can, I can, and I'm going to do it." For Norma, being "mother and father" means providing both emotional and economic care for her children as a single parent. Thus, facing Manlo's abandonment, Norma makes her own sacrifice and assumes the responsibilities of caring for her children and continuing family life in his absence. This mirrors how Norma responds to her daughter María José's migration years later, as Norma again assumes primary caregiving responsibility for the child of a migrant parent, this time becoming "mother and father" for her grandson Jeremy. Across generations, Norma shares in the sacrifice of transnational migration—even as she herself does not leave Nicaragua—by assuming responsibilities for children's care and by making sense of the disruptions of migration by drawing on values for unity and sacrifice to regenerate family life.

Somewhat distinctly from Norma, Angela frames her husband's migration unequivocally in terms of abandonment. Carlo left for the United States in 1989, at the end of the Sandinista Revolutionary period, when Nicaragua faced social and economic instability as a result of the US-funded Contra war and embargo.[9] Angela was left to raise four young children on her own. Carlo migrated for economic reasons, and joined thousands of Nicaraguans immigrating to the United States during the late 1980s. Given US geopolitical hostility toward the Sandinista regime, Nicaraguans who settled in the United States during this period were eventually able to apply for legal residency.[10]

Angela was generally supportive of her husband's emigration at first, viewing migration as needed to improve her family's economic circumstances. She recalls that Carlo left with the "*sueño*" (dream) of greater economic opportunity and with the promise that he would share this opportunity with his family in Nicaragua. She remembers him promising her, "We would get ahead, our children would get a better education, that he was going to do something for us." However, this dream of migration was shattered within six months, as Carlo stopped sending remittances home and as his communication with his family in Nicaragua became increasingly infrequent. Angela eventually found out that he was living with another woman with whom he shared a household and whom he eventually married—without first divorcing Angela." Years of division, conflict, and mistrust in the family followed, as Angela's eldest daughter, Noelia, blamed Angela for Carlo's departure and as her sons aligned with her against Carlo. This experience continues to cast a shadow over Angela's view of migration, for she squarely attributes the division within her family—between herself, her husband, and her children—to migration. As Angela puts it, "Why did all of this happen? Because he left, because he migrated . . . If he hadn't left, all these things wouldn't have happened."

More important in reinforcing Angela's sense of migration as abandonment than even her feelings of personal betrayal are Carlo's failed promises to support their children. When Angela's daughter and son (Karla and Jonathan) left for Miami in the 1990s, Carlo refused to let them stay in his house. (According to Angela, his new wife didn't want his adult children from a previous marriage living with them.) Further, even though Carlo eventually obtained legal residency status in the United States, he refused to use his legal status to help petition for his children, leaving them to negotiate life in the United States as undocumented migrants, facing dangers and insecurities Angela viewed as unnecessary (and provoked by their father's abandonment). For Angela, then, migration is tinged by disillusionment and by her sense that migration's ultimate end is a severing of responsibilities to family members back home. This experience of migration as abandonment casts a shadow across Angela's views of migration in subsequent generations.

The Second Generation: Migration as Sacrifice

Even though both women share past experiences of husbands' migrations as abandonments, Angela and Norma attempt to frame their daughters' migrations as necessary sacrifices. Situating mother migration as a sacrifice made for the sake of children opens the space for grandmothers to participate in what is construed as the shared, intergenerational sacrifice of migration. In this narrative framing, women who migrate sacrifice by working abroad and sending remittances home to support children's care. Women who assume primary caregiving responsibilities also sacrifice, as mothers supporting migrant daughters and as grandmothers raising grandchildren. In other words, women participate in the shared sacrifice of migration across generations and over borders, even as they themselves may not migrate. However, while the migration as sacrifice narrative helps family members make sense of the distance and time that characterize transnational life, the counter narrative of migration as abandonment is ever-present, carried from a prior generation and threatening to undo the ties of relationality that grandmothers stitch together through their caregiving.

As mothers, Angela and Norma have worried about the safety, security, and well-being of their migrant children, worries exacerbated by their children's initial undocumented status. Migrant mothers Karla (Angela's daughter) and Mariá José (Norma's daughter) experienced difficulties related to lack of legal documentation, especially during their first years in the United States, as they sought steady employment, housing, and security. These challenges were felt back home in Nicaragua, as Norma and Angela worried about their daughters' welfare and had to get by without the regular support of remittances (which would come later). Further, both Angela and Norma were frustrated that their migrant children did not receive the support that their fathers had promised. However, where Norma's response to the hardships her migrant daughters faced was one of ongoing encouragement and support, Angela remained more reticent about migration and its repercussions on her family.[12]

María José migrated to the United States in 2000 at the age of eighteen, leaving her son Jeremy, one year old at the time, in Norma's care. María José's sister Vanesa had emigrated a year before, in 1999, at the age of nineteen; Vanesa did not have any children at the time. María José traveled to the United States alone, but hoped to meet with her sister and their father in Miami. While María José and Vanesa both left Nicaragua with plans to rejoin their father in Miami, Manlo's lack of support pushed María José in particular to consider whether to stay in the United States or whether to return to her son in Nicaragua.

As María José faced the pending expiration of her tourist visa, she shared her uncertainty about returning to Nicaragua with her mother. Norma recalls the telephone call she received from María José (who she calls "Mary"), as she sought advice at that pivotal moment in her migration journey:

> She asked me, "Mommy, what do I do now?" This was after a month there. I told her, "Mary," honestly I told her, "Mary, don't come back. Stay there. Do it for your son."
>
> "But," she told me, "I miss my baby." I told her, "Mary, stay there, your baby is in good hands. I am going to turn him over to you healthy and safe. Work, apply yourself, because in Nicaragua nothing good awaits you. You're young, you can start a different life there, you have opportunities that Nicaragua can't offer you. Stay and fight, do it for your son."
>
> That's how I took on the great responsibility of raising Jeremy.

Norma's recollection of this conversation clearly situates migration within the frame of sacrifice. As a mother, she encouraged her daughter to stay in the United States and to take advantage of the opportunities she would have there, even if it meant missing her son; in fact, according to Norma, María José should view migration as a sacrifice made for the sake of her son. Norma situates herself in this intergenerational story of mother migration and sacrifice, as she supports her migrant daughter by taking on the "great responsibility" of raising her grandson. In other words, as a mother of a migrant daughter, Norma too participates in the sacrifice of migration, even though she herself does not cross national borders; caregiving is her intergenerational sacrifice.

Central to the way Norma frames her role within her transnational family is that she has been "mother and father" for her grandson after his mother emigrated, just as she was for her children upon their father's emigration a generation before. Norma foregrounds the personal sacrifices that grandmothering entails, describing how she focused her energy and attention on raising Jeremy rather than pursuing her personal aspirations for career advancement or relational intimacy in later adult life. Even as Norma is clear about the "*dolor y sufrimiento*" (pain and suffering) of raising her grandson following mother migration, she also describes grandmothering as "one of the most marvelous things that could have happened to me." Norma has enjoyed a close and "special" relationship with Jeremy over the years, in part because mothering in a second generation has given her more "emotional maturity" from which to draw in raising Jeremy. Norma also frames grandmothering in relation to the intergenerational cycle of migration in which the values of sacrifice and care are regenerated in her family. Norma says she is concluding this cycle of familial migration and regeneration with her grandson: "With Jeremy I'm closing [the cycle]." In this way, Norma is also alluding to a future where Jeremy will rejoin his mother abroad, bringing to an end the cycle of migration and care that has shaped much of Norma's adult life.

Central to Norma's care of Jeremy is how she draws upon the narrative of migration as sacrifice to help Jeremy make sense of his mother's migration. Throughout the ten years of María José's absence, Norma has reiterated to Jeremy that she is his grandmother, that his mother lives in the United States, and that María José's absence is necessary for his welfare. For instance, Norma recounts how when Jeremy was a young child, she would show him photographs of María José and put the phone to his ear, telling him, "*Ella es tu mamá*" (She's your mother). Norma also made sure that María José communicated with Jeremy frequently, and would remind her grandson after every phone call that his mother was working hard in the United States for his benefit.[13] For ten years, Norma has engaged in the transnational kin work of maintaining the mother-child tie by teaching Jeremy to identify María José as his mother, regularly communicate with her, and, most importantly, to respect the sacrifices María José makes for him. By extension, Norma figures herself into this transnational story of care and sacrifice, as she is the caregiver simultaneously responsible for her grandson and for upholding the mother-child relationship, receding into the background as she actively foregrounds her grandson's relationship with his migrant mother.

who longs to share physical copresence with her mother and who increasingly questions the purpose of her mother's ongoing absence from her life. Previously a top student, at eleven years old, Laleska's grades began to fall, and her teachers reached out to Angela to signal their concerns. Angela, trying to motivate her granddaughter to improve her school performance, reminded her, "Your mom is over there working hard. Don't think that they just *give* her money; it demands a lot of hard work. You have to take advantage of her hard work; you *have* to study." In this framing, studying hard and doing well at school becomes Laleska's obligation within her transnational family; succeeding at school is a way for grandchildren to participate in the shared intergenerational sacrifice of migration. Nonetheless, this message didn't seem to reach Laleska, who continued to refuse to talk with Karla when she telephoned from Miami. When I asked Laleska why she didn't like to talk on the phone with her mother, she replied, "What good is it all if she's not here with me? If I don't have her here with me?" In her own way, Laleska was pushing back against the framing of her mother's migration as a necessary sacrifice, presenting a counter narrative emerging from her feelings of distance and abandonment. This dynamic demonstrates how narrative frames of migration are relational; narratives are formed, shared, or contested within families, as family members engage with the often-troublesome realities of transnational life. In Laleska's case, her growing sense of emotional distance from her migrant mother mirrors Angela's experience of her husband's abandonment decades earlier, revealing how the narrative of migration as abandonment reverberates and accumulates significance across time, shaping responses to migration over generations.

Angela witnesses the growing distance between Karla and Laleska and responds by encouraging her daughter to offset this gap by calling and visiting with more regularity. However, even as Angela's kin work seeks to hold mother and child together, it is challenged by the realities of transnational life. For instance, the fact that Karla has three US-born children means her emotional energy is divided across borders, leaving Laleska to feel as though she receives less attention than her mother's coresident children. Further, time itself acts in ways that lend toward feelings of abandonment; in Angela's words, "Time . . . time is separating us and separating us." Angela's efforts to uphold a close tie between Karla and Laleska are an attempt to remake the past through the present, to help prevent Laleska from experiencing the abandonment that Angela experienced, first as a wife and then as a mother. Such intergenerational kin work struggles to offset the effects of time and distance, to uphold relational ties and family values in transnational families. However, given Angela's past experiences, the possibility of loss remains ever present, tainting transnational intimacies with the threat of abandonment.

For their part, Norma and Jeremy seem unequivocally positive about Jeremy's future migration to join his mother in the United States. The narrative of sacrifice that Norma has reiterated over time forms a central theme of her transnational caregiving; it is a narrative that encourages Jeremy to look forward to rejoining his mother abroad. Norma has encouraged María José to weather the difficulties of migrant life abroad, giving Norma an even stronger stake in the success of her daughter's migration trajectory. Similarly, Norma has encouraged Jeremy to view his mother's migration as a sacrifice made for his benefit. This helps explain Jeremy's positive outlook toward his mother's migration; he continually emphasizes that, "She is working over there so I can go to school over here." Jeremy is also focused on what he and Norma view as his pending reunification with María José. In Jeremy's account of his mother's migration, she "went away to process my paperwork [residency visa]. The sooner she left, the sooner she would come back. That's why I wasn't sad." Jeremy would discuss his concrete plans for rejoining his mother, who lived in New York, saying he was ready to buy winter clothing and acclimate to the cold climate. While Jeremy acknowledged he would be "a little sad" to leave his grandmother, he talked about visiting her frequently in the future. In short, Jeremy faced his reunification with his mother with confidence, reflecting the positive orientation of more than ten years of Norma's caregiving.

Jeremy's reunion with his mother in the United States was a culmination of María José's and Norma's past sacrifices, as migrant mother and caregiving grandmother. Both Norma and María José told me they had reiterated to Jeremy that reunification was the goal of María José's migration ever since he was old enough to ask questions about her migration. Norma recalls how María José would repeat to Jeremy in their phone calls and internet-based conversations, "One day we're going to be together; you're going to see that everything's going to be all right." For her part, Norma would tell Jeremy, "You have to be with your mom one day. You have to pray to God so that your mom can legalize her status and come get you so that you have an opportunity that you don't have here in Nicaragua." Norma acknowledges she will miss Jeremy a great deal when he leaves Nicaragua, just as she missed her daughter years before. However, she views her emotional pain as a further sacrifice she will make for her transnational family. As Norma sees it, "Of course, I'm going to miss him, but it's another necessary sacrifice so that he can be with his mother and so that they can have a better life."

María José had not visited Nicaragua until 2010 when she returned for a two-week visit (during which I had an opportunity to meet and briefly interview her). I interviewed Norma a week before María José's visit, and found her and Jeremy visibly excited with anticipation. According to Norma, María José's intention was to take Jeremy back to the United States with her; she had told Norma that Jeremy's visa was processed and that all that remained was to obtain his Nicaraguan passport so he could fly back to the United States with her. As it turned out, María José's visit did not unfold as planned. In their interview with immigration officials at the US Embassy, Norma and María José were informed that some aspects of the family reunification visa petition for Jeremy remained incomplete. As a result, Jeremy would be unable to enter the United States at that time. Although Norma told me that she, María José, and Jeremy were all disappointed by this news, María José herself tried to cast her visit in a positive frame by reaffirming her commitment to bring Jeremy to the United States with her one day, hopefully soon.

Whereas Norma draws on a narrative of migration as sacrifice to orient Jeremy positively toward his pending reunification with his mother, Angela and Laleska are much more ambivalent about Laleska's possible emigration. When Angela talks about Laleska perhaps rejoining her mother in Miami, a foreboding sense of abandonment comes across in her narrative. For instance, Angela emphasizes that Laleska has grown accustomed to *her* care, and wonders how she will react to the care of her "mamá Karla," whether she will learn to respect her mother after more than a decade of separation, and how she will adapt to living with her new stepfather and half siblings. Angela's concerns are exacerbated by what she perceives as the growing emotional distance between Karla and Laleska that has emerged over recent years. Without a visit from Karla, in the face of Laleska's deepening reluctance to communicate with her mother, Angela feels increasingly unable to bridge a growing mother-daughter divide. Further, as Laleska feels increasingly separated from her "mother Karla," Angela finds herself feeling increasingly separated from her daughter, unable to persuade Karla of what she views as the looming possibility that her migration may end in abandonment. In Angela's words, *"Lo que sienta ella, siento yo"* (What she [Laleska] feels, I feel).

Unlike Jeremy, who looks forward to talking with his mother on a daily basis using cell phone and internet technology, Laleska often resisted the overtures to communicate made by Karla from abroad. For instance, Laleska refused to come to the phone when her mother called and made excuses to avoid internet-based conversations. Laleska told me that she viewed communication with Karla as futile, "Because why does it serve me, to talk to her, if she isn't here by my side to help me?" Laleska's refusal to communicate with her mother seems to reflect her growing emotional distance with Karla. In response, Angela encourages Laleska to recognize and appreciate the sacrifices her mother makes for her benefit. Nonetheless, the narrative of migration as sacrifice cannot contain Laleska's growing sense of abandonment, which threatens to undo Angela's attempts to regenerate family life.

As these examples illustrate, the possibility of children's reunification with mothers abroad poses a challenge to the framing of migration as sacrifice, reminding both grandmothers and children of the possibility of abandonment. On one hand, central to a grandmother's care and kin work is upholding the emotional relationships between migrant mothers and their children over transnational space and time. And yet, although grandmothers assume the responsibility for children's care and grow emotionally close to their grandchildren in the process, grandmothers must relinquish these ties when faced with the possibility of mother-child reunification. Rather than frame the potential future separation from their grandchildren as a form of abandonment, however, grandmothers may situate their support of reunification as another means of personally participating in the shared sacrifice of migration. In other words, grandmothers' support of mother-child reunification can be framed within the sacrifice narrative: grandmothers put aside the physical and emotional closeness they have attained with their grandchildren over years of caregiving and sacrifice their personal desires for the sake of unity and togetherness in family relations.

Conclusion: Narratives as Intergenerational Care

Fostering and sustaining narratives of migration over generations is central to the kin work of grandmother caregivers in transnational families. Narratives help make meaning out of the disruptions and uncertainties of migration, but they are also fragile and contested by family members, across generations, in response to the tensions of transnational life. In Nicaraguan transnational families, two narrative frames shift back and forth over time, sustained by family members' actions, responses, and experiences of migration: migration as sacrifice and migration as abandonment. As the stories of Norma and Angela demonstrate, understanding the effects of migration on families requires a perspective that foregrounds temporality, that is, how migration shapes family life over time and across generations. Grandmother caregivers create narratives to render significance from previous experiences of their husbands' migrations, framing the meaning of their adult daughters' migrations, and helping guide their grandchildren's orientations toward the possibility of their future migrations. In this way, a narrative analysis of transnational family life weaves together past, present, and future and thus highlights the tensions that emerge over time within kin relationships reconfigured across transnational space and time. Broadening our perspective on transnational family life by attending to the care work and kin work accomplished by women of the grandmother generation in migrant-sending families is an important way to move beyond a biological mother-child or nuclear family conceptualization of transnational families. Furthermore, foregrounding narratives casts grandmothers as agents within global migration processes even though they themselves do not cross national borders.

Narratives are central to intergenerational kin work, as they assist children, mothers, and grandmothers in making sense of the disjunctures between cultural expectations for family life and the ways care and kinship are reconfigured in the context of global migration. The analysis presented here reconstructs migration narratives as they are framed and contested across what I have described as three generations of migration within two Nicaraguan transnational families. Of course, this analysis would be enhanced by tracing family histories back in time—for instance, documenting the processes through which families settled in the capital city in previous generations—and following children forward and analyzing how their possible reunification with mothers abroad reconfigures care and kin relations into the future. Even within the scope of the present analysis, however, a narrative approach on transnational family life enhances our understandings of women's care and kin work over time. Across the generations, caregivers and other family members shift between narratives of sacrifice and abandonment, attempting to render significance from the threats to anticipated life courses posed by migration. In the face of these threats, care is not just about social reproduction, but about regeneration, responding to disruptions in family life—to the changes and challenges of transnational migration—by fostering cultural values over time and across generations.

ACKNOWLEDGMENTS

Many thanks to Cati Coe and Parin Dossa for inviting me to participate in this collection and for their helpful comments on earlier drafts of this chapter. Thank you to the Care and the Lifecourse writing group (Elana Buch, Laura Heinemann, Julia Kowalski, Jessica Robbins-Roszkowski, and Aaron Seaman) for ongoing support and critical feedback on my thinking and writing about care. The field research upon which this chapter is based was supported by the National Science Foundation and the Fulbright Institute for International Education. At the University of Oregon, I am grateful for the support of the Underrepresented Minority Retention Program and the Oregon Humanities Center.

NOTES

1. Perhaps best summarized by Arlene Geronimus through her work on "weathering," research shows that for African American women in particular, health status at midlife reflects an embodied accumulation of social hardships associated with racial discrimination across the life course (Geronimus et al. 2006).
2. Although grandmother caregiving in Nicaragua is not unique to families of migrants, what is distinct about intergenerational care in transnational families is that grandmothers must respond to the challenges posed by prolonged absence, distance, and fraying emotional ties.

3. All names used here are pseudonyms.

4. In the wake of their husbands' migrations, Norma and Angela were left raising four children each as single mothers.

5. Both Jeremy and Laleska also attend semiprivate schools, showing the importance of education in families of migrants. Private school tuition at the time of the study was 75 córdobas/month, 2.50 in US dollars.

6. There are two main political parties in Nicaragua: the FSLN, or Sandinistas, and the PLC, Partido Liberal Constitucional (Liberal Constitutional Party), which remains the main opposition to the FSLN and continues to receive U.S. political support.

7. Because of US hostility toward the Sandinista regime, US policy was to accept migrants like Manlo during this period as "political refugees," and offer them asylum and legal paths to US residency. For more on US geopolitics toward Central America in the 1980s and 1990s and its impact on immigration policy, see Susan Bibler Coutin (2005).

8. Norma describes how several Nicaraguan women became leaders in this clandestine crossing of food into Nicaragua in the 1980s, as they would purchase powdered milk in Honduras and sell it back home. She says, "So in that way we organized ourselves and thus overcame many things, and for that reason my children are alive."

9. For an excellent overview of this period of US intervention in Nicaragua's political and economic affairs, see the Introduction to Roger Lancaster's 1992 ethnography, *Life Is Hard.*

10. Seven years after the Contra war ended, the US Congress passed the 1997 Nicaraguan and Central American Adjustment and Relief Act (NACARA), which granted residency to some 55,000 Nicaraguans who had entered the country prior to December 1, 1995.

11. This threw Angela into a years-long legal limbo, as she needed to determine his marital status abroad in order to file for divorce in Nicaragua, and needed Carlo's signature on divorce paperwork in order to assume the title to their house in Managua.

12. Two of Angela's other children, Carlo and Noelia, also have migration experience: Carlo migrated to the United States with a student visa in 1995 and studied for two years in a post-baccalaureate program in a public university before returning to Nicaragua. Noelia left for Costa Rica with a boyfriend in the mid-1990s and subsequently (within a year) returned to Nicaragua. She attempted migration again in 2004, this time to the United States (several years after her siblings Karla and Jonathan had settled in Miami). Noelia's journey through Mexico en route to the United States is a harrowing tale of danger and ultimately she was detained by U.S. Border Patrol and held at a federal detention facility for more than a month before being deported back to Nicaragua. Norma's daughter Vanesa emigrated a year before María José on a tourist visa, and also stayed beyond its expiration. Vanesa has since obtained legal permanent residency in the United States. Although space limits me from further analyzing migration experiences of Angela and Norma's other children, these brief details hint at the complex circumstances shaping family members' relationship to, and narratives of, migration.

13. During the first eight years of María José's migration, this communication occurred via telephone, but over the last two years, Jeremy has spoken to his mother using an Internet connection and desktop computer purchased with María José's remittances. Young Jeremy has become adept at managing different software programs and social networking sites in order to "chat" with his "mamá María."

14. Although Angela overcame this earlier episode of depression, she relives similar feelings of sadness through her granddaughter's emotional reaction to her mother's migration. For instance, after Karla's visit to Nicaragua years before came to an end,

Angela remembers Laleska crying, and she recalls, "I felt her sadness too." In this way, the emotional response to mother migration is transgenerational, transpersonal, and transnational (also see Horton 2009).

15. In Nicaragua, "evangelical" refers to a non-Catholic Christian. Norma and Angela regularly attend church services and both have held leadership positions in their respective churches.

16. I discuss women's emotional responses to migration, caregiving reconfigurations, and transnational family life in detail in Kristin Elizabeth Yarris (2014a).

17. I describe the benefits and inadequacies of remittances from children's perspectives more fully in Yarris (2014b).

PART TWO

Reconfigurations of Kinship and Care in Migration Contexts

4

Fostering Change

Elderly Foster Mothers' Intergenerational Influence in Contemporary China

ERIN L. RAFFETY

Auntie Ma, the foster mother of eleven-year-old Meili, was also the mother of an only daughter who had recently married, moved in with her in-laws, and begun the process of starting a family of her own.[1] Although Auntie Ma's biological daughter also lived in the capital city of Nanning, she saw her infrequently, and she was unlikely to provide her any practical or physical support in old age given Guangxi's[2] traditional patterns of patrilocal residence.[3] Auntie Ma was also a widow, who received a small monthly pension from the state. She lived alone in a seventh-story apartment, and her extended family lived many hours away in the countryside. Hence, like many elderly in China, Auntie Ma was vulnerable due to her relative familial and social marginality, her limited finances, and her lack of social networks.

However, over the course of my fieldwork, I discovered that despite her frequent and humble self-critique of her own simple background and uneducated status, Auntie Ma did not represent herself as a victim of her circumstances. She spoke notably, openly, and brazenly about hardships during the Cultural Revolution.[4] Although she bemoaned how her youth was taken away from her when she was sent to the rice paddies in Longzhou, close to the Vietnam and Yunnan borders, and mourned the early death of her husband, she, like many other foster mothers, was remarkably generous, resourceful, and kind.

The last time I saw Auntie Ma she shoved a bulging bag of peanuts she had brought back from the countryside into my purse, and insisted on walking me, as she always did, across the six-lane highway to the bus stop. She began to talk about how she felt quite lucky in her life given her circumstances: growing up in poverty with her family, who had only one pair of shoes to share among five children; living through the Cultural Revolution and the Great Leap Forward;

and recalling all those who had died or now had no insurance or pension. I remember very clearly as we stood by the side of the crowded road, traffic rushing by, exhaust pouring out of the noisy buses, that she looked quite content when she said that she knew from experience that she was living in the best times in China and she did not take it for granted. She remarked poignantly that now that her foster daughter Meili was about to be adopted to America, she felt she'd done at least one thing right with her life and could die a happy woman.

Filial Piety, Intergenerational Contracts, and Social Change

Across the Asian world, scholars note the waning of filial piety and the rise of youth culture, conjugal intimacy, and market capitalism, which is leaving seniors politically, economically, and socially vulnerable. This is particularly significant in China, where the all-encompassing virtue of filial piety—the respect, devotion, and care for one's elders and ancestors, which once undergirded social life—seems to be fading (Ikels 2004). However, the chapters in this volume, and other recent scholarship, including my own work with foster families, suggest such demographic and cultural shifts are not so clear cut. Not only do global demographic trends surprisingly point to the prevailing, yet somewhat hidden, importance of grandparents to social reproduction in modernity (Chen, Lu, and Mair 2011; Settles et al. 2009), but scholars of China (and across Asia; see, for instance, Khan and Kobayashi, this volume) are also recognizing that filial piety might not be so much dead as being reinterpreted and renegotiated (Croll 2006; Zhang 2004).

My fieldwork with elderly Chinese foster mothers shows that even as such seniors find themselves economically, politically, and socially disadvantaged, their kin work as foster parents to abandoned, disabled children (most of whom are eventually adopted internationally) provides them certain economic, political, and social recuperation. Perhaps most surprisingly, my ethnographic fieldwork, conducted over eighteen months between 2010 and 2012 in the Guangxi Autonomous Region, shows that foster mothers are not merely reacting to shifting family patterns and their own insecurity, but are also challenging middle-aged orphanage staff and international governmental organization (INGO) care workers' notions of child-rearing and family. Yet, literature regarding the reinterpretation of filial piety in the Asian world, as well as literature on migration (as Dossa and Coe note in their introduction to this volume), has been substantially biased toward the perspective of youth as the site of social change. Hence, I aim to critique and refine such literature by demonstrating that far from being merely vulnerable or burdensome, senior foster mothers' adaptation in transnational kinship actually places them at the center of social change.

In this chapter, I first demonstrate that the literature on the elderly in Asia stresses the vulnerability of these seniors in the face of population growth, lack of state pension, and the breakdown of traditional cultural logics and structures of filial piety. Next, I argue that despite an emerging literature that examines the persistence of the intergenerational contract in Asia and its reciprocal reinterpretation by both seniors and their middle-generation children, such literature still positions seniors as primarily reacting to changing youth attitudes rather than influencing family culture. I posit that by looking at elderly foster mothers like Auntie Ma, who are abandoned by their middle-aged biological children and take in nonbiological, disabled, abandoned foster children, we might see alternative strategies of rehabilitative kin work in Chinese society.

In the sections that follow, I draw upon my fieldwork with Chinese foster families in Guangxi to demonstrate that elderly women's vulnerability becomes a resource that repositions them as uniquely open to receiving abandoned, disabled children. The bonds that develop between them and their foster children lend themselves to economic, social, and political rehabilitation. By foregrounding the intergenerational conflicts between middle-aged orphanage and INGO care workers regarding the elderly foster mothers' motivations to foster, I highlight the contentious nature of this kin work. I show how the intergenerational relationships between foster mothers and foster children encroach upon the insecurities of middle-aged INGO and orphanage personnel, causing them to envy the very families they seek to control. In illuminating this reversal of intergenerational influence, I suggest that the reinterpretation of filial piety in China has been too quick to assume that seniors are merely recipients or adaptors, rather than instigators, of social change (Croll 2006; Li 2009; Qi 2014; Zhang 2005).

Elderly Abandonment and Vulnerability in China

Many scholars have noted the significant vulnerability for Asia's rapidly growing elderly populations given shifting cultural practices, increasing economic pressures, and scant state welfare. Perhaps nowhere else in the Asian world has social change been as dramatic for the elderly as in China, where nearly sixty million people who came of age during the Communist Revolution, toiled in the countryside, and lived and breathed socialist rhetoric, quickly found themselves struggling to catch up with modern education, entrepreneurship, and open markets (Yan 2010). Indeed, such elderly were unable to take advantage of the economic reforms of the 1980s because they were implemented after or as they retired. Meanwhile, the disintegration of the collective economy that made old-age support almost entirely the responsibility of family members, the collapse of supporting structures for the institution of filial piety, and the lack of effective intervention mechanisms for parental neglect makes China's elderly particularly vulnerable (Zhang 2004, 84). For rural seniors especially, the lack of pension for farmers makes them almost entirely reliant on family members for care in old age. For all seniors, the early mandatory retirement ages in China (age fifty-five for women and sixty for men) often robs elderly of their earning abilities and of their social status with regard to their power in family decision making as well as their position in the wider society. According to the 2010 census, at 178 million, today's elders over the age of sixty make up 13.3 percent of the population, but they are projected to make up nearly 30 percent of China's total population by 2050.

Hong Zhang, in her work on elderly abandonment in China, and Xiaoyuan Shang and Xiaoming Wu, in their work on social welfare, have shown that China's elderly constitute some of the most exposed members of contemporary society, because the familial system of generational caregiving is breaking down, especially across increasing distance and failing extended family bonds (Shang and Wu 2011; Zhang 2004, 2005). To many, this is as much evidence of shifting economic and demographic circumstances as it is testament to the waning cultural value that elders have in contemporary society. As Yunxiang Yan first argued in *Private Life under Socialism* (2003), since the post-Mao era, the conjugal unit has triumphed, and the elderly have lost their financial security, as well as familial and social functions and status. No longer operating as heads of the household within the family or publicly within the village community, patriarchy in its historical and traditional sense in China has all but disappeared. Yan has also been particularly critical of a certain immorality and incivility that he registers ethnographically among China's youth, whose market-driven individualist attitudes cause them to renege on obligations to their elders (2003, 2011a, 2011b). The Chinese government, which in many ways effectively undermined this cultural system of patriarchy and filial piety under socialism (Yan 2003), shirks responsibility for the growing elderly population, however, at the same time ensuring by law children's obligation to care for their parents in old age.[5]

Notable counterpoints to Yan's charges of incivility, the rise of individuality, and the death of patriarchy are exemplified by the work of Elizabeth J. Croll (2006), Hongshi Li (2009), Xiaoying Qi (2014), and Hong Zhang (2005), which emphasizes that middle and senior generations are actually maintaining, yet simultaneously reinterpreting intergenerational contracts. These scholars argue that in response to new patterns of family, production, and migration initiated by middle-aged children, elders are maneuvering to ensure their old age security by providing inheritance, housing, and childcare to children. However, despite the contention that filial piety is being reinterpreted reciprocally by contemporary families, these scholars nonetheless position seniors as *responding* to their middle-aged children rather than influencing intergenerational change. For instance, when Hongshi Li (2009) describes changes in the gendered practice of filial piety in northeastern China, she highlights the shifting expectation of young men and women's marriage practices and inheritance. In other words, parents are willing to provide sizeable monetary gifts in life (rather than after death) in order to ensure that their children will support them in old age. Likewise, with the exception of the self-reliance strategy mentioned by Hong Zhang among aging parents, seniors are portrayed as adopting "active coping strategies," which respond to modern birth control policies and increasing demands for economic investment in their children's futures (2005, 62).

Therefore, despite illuminating the reciprocal nature of the intergenerational contract in contemporary Asia, scholars such as Croll, Li, Qi, and Zhang nonetheless depict Chinese elders' actions and attitudes as responses and reactions to the influence of the middle generation. With the exception of Zhang, these scholars' research primarily considers the Asian family as a closed, biological unit rather than acknowledging other manifestations of the family that may develop primarily from the breakdown of the biological family unit under the stress of modernity. Alongside others in this section who note novel reconfigurations of contemporary kinship (for instance Loretta Baldassar's exploration of the impact of polymedia communications on caregiving in this volume), in this chapter, I consider how kin work among elderly foster mothers and their nonbiological foster children might challenge these contemporary arguments about the directions and dynamics of intergenerational change in intergenerational relationships in China. Why do elderly foster mothers take in abandoned, disabled children? If they are abandoned by their own biological families and the state, how do their actions reposition them? Simply put: Is elderly foster care primarily a reactive strategy to vulnerable circumstances or does it foster social change?

Foster Care and Fieldwork

The height of foster care practices coincided with the Temporary Policy on Foster Care issued by the Communist Party in late 2003 and extended until the peak year for international adoptions from China in 2005. Although by this time foster care had been established as a strategy of poor orphanages to compensate for scarcity of caregivers, as well as a strategy for rich, urban orphanages to ready children for international adoption, the policy officially mandated the development and participation of state orphanages in foster care projects. It also clarified the terms of the arrangements: foster parents were to have ample space and an income commensurate with the local average, be between the ages of thirty-five and sixty-five, and possess the time and the abilities to care for children (Wu, Han, and Gao 2005). In exchange for their services foster parents were paid a monthly stipend commensurate with local standards of living, but children remained wards of the state until they were returned to the orphanage or adopted.

Gradually, such placements became lucrative for state orphanages that could receive sizeable foreign donations in exchange for these children once China opened to international adoption in the mid-1990s. Even though international adoptions of healthy babies from China have dropped dramatically since the mid-2000s, a disproportionate number of children with disabilities in the Chinese state orphanage system are still being primarily adopted to the West. According to recent statistics, special needs children comprise more than half of all US-China adoptions today (Crary 2010), and this number may be much higher given that state social welfare institutions across China boast special needs populations of nearly 80 to 90 percent (Hu and Szente 2009). Although abandonment of children with special needs in rural areas has historically been higher (and the strain on less resourced institutions is substantially more severe), a steady and climbing stream of children are also being abandoned in China's modern cities. While sociologist Leslie Wang (2010) concludes that this abandonment of children with disabilities testifies to increasingly market-driven attitudes of China's middle generation, Xiaoyuan Shang's (2008) work on kin adoption and my own work in Guangxi suggests that motivations for disabled child abandonment have significant social roots.

Not unlike for the elderly, the Chinese government provides little financial, structural, or social welfare for children with disabilities, relying substantially on the family unit to provide expensive and comprehensive care for such children (Shang and Fisher 2013). Under modern birth planning policies, safeguards such as kin fosterage that served to divide and provide care for vulnerable or over-quota children are now less prominent given shrinking family size (especially in urban areas), widespread migration that makes family members unavailable to provide care, and cultural shifts away from patriarchy, extended families, and intergenerational caregiving. However, as children are still perceived in terms of their broader social worth, their ability to provide care in old age for their parents and their ability to fulfill social familial roles, children with disabilities present a particular strain on the family unit. Their impairments render them not only economically and physically, but also socially vulnerable, because if they cannot provide for their parents or participate in society, they are considered effectively "non-human" (Guo and Kleinman 2011).

Because of their precarious place in modern Chinese social life, children with disabilities have not only been abandoned with great frequency, but are often sequestered away from society in state orphanages on the outskirts of sprawling cities. In my initial forays into fieldwork, I struggled to gain access to state orphanages that were suspicious of foreigners looking to expose poor conditions for children with disabilities in China's welfare homes. After approximately six months of building relationships with INGOs, officials, and orphanages in 2010, I was finally allowed into the municipal orphanage in early 2011 to conduct official research. This relationship was largely brokered by an INGO, Mercy Care, that worked closely with the state orphanage foster care program in Guangxi and took me under its wing. Although I eventually gained unlimited access to foster families in the state orphanage program, I was not permitted to videotape or tape-record interviews within the orphanage or with foster families in their homes and had to rely on handwritten notes to re-create my interactions and conversations with informants.

Although to some extent these precautions reflect the sensitive nature of my research, given that most of the children in foster care were abandoned and disabled, they also illuminated some significant demographics and tensions reflected in these foster care relationships. I quickly discovered that contrary to my initial hypotheses, foster parents were by and large elderly, the majority over age fifty-five, and many over sixty-five, despite national regulations. When I questioned the orphanage and INGO monitors, all of whom where between the ages of twenty-five and forty-five, about this, they were embarrassed and apologetic, stating that they could not find anyone else willing to foster disabled, abandoned children for the meager stipend the orphanage provided. A puzzle emerged in my fieldwork: although elderly foster parents were somewhat perfectly positioned to foster given their solitary lives and scant finances, they were also highly scrutinized by middle-aged orphanage and INGO monitors for these very reasons. Why were the features that at once motivated elderly women to foster so highly suspicious and problematic to their middle-aged counterparts? I suggest that the provision of foster care did not constitute mere kin work that intervened to fill a social void. Rather I found that such caregiving was highly contested, imbued with the vulnerabilities and insecurities of not just poor, elderly women, but also middle-aged government actors.

Social Vulnerability as a Resource

Elderly foster parents with whom I did fieldwork were both practically impoverished and socially marginalized. As I chatted with foster families in the villages, or even in the regional capital, the story was always the same. These foster parents' grown children had migrated to bustling cities to find work in factories, and depending on how far away, they returned on the weekends, monthly, or just once a year. In a society in which children are meant to care for their parents in old age (Potter and Potter 1990), many elderly, despite fulfilling their sociocultural obligations to their children and society, found themselves physically and/or emotionally abandoned by children or other relatives who had left them behind to forge a future in more prosperous cities.

However, when questioned directly about their motivations to foster, elderly foster parents candidly weighed differential and emergent reasons, crafting a narrative that reflected their awareness regarding both their social vulnerability and the substantial social benefits they gained from fostering. For instance, when Auntie Ma spoke about her decision to foster, her narrative reflected multiple motivations that developed and shifted over time. Like many other parents, through observation of neighbors' experiences, Auntie Ma gradually became interested in fostering:

> Well, you know my neighbors had fostered children, and I became curious. And I thought, to have a child, you know, I could do that, it's just me, and the government doesn't pay me much in retirement, so I also thought of the money. And so I had one child, and she had to go back to the orphanage. But by that point I was used to having her around, and then I took in Meili, and she's been with me for six years. And you develop feelings you know, you want more for them, like me, what can I give her, really? Of course, I love her, but I want an American mother to adopt her to give her everything she deserves.

Auntie Ma's rationale for why she chose to foster begins with the motivation of curiosity. Next she mentions her (presumably physical and emotional) ability to do so, alongside the financial incentive of fostering a child. Additionally she comments on the experience of "getting used to having a child around." Finally, she expresses the development of feelings for her foster daughter, Meili, and her desire to give her a better life.

Not unlike Yuping Wu, Xiaoyu Han, and Qin Gao in their book on foster care in urban Beijing (2005), I also found that foster parents' motivations for fostering were multiple, overlapping, and emergent. However, I want to suggest that for women like Auntie Ma, their social vulnerability, a presumed disadvantage of their circumstances, was a primary motivator in their acceptance and raising of abandoned, disabled children. Indeed, following her assertion of curiosity, the intermingling in the phrasing of Auntie Ma's motivations is highly significant. When she states, "to have a child, you know, I could do that, it's just me, and the government doesn't pay me much in retirement, so I also thought of the money," her social vulnerability is certainly apparent, but also subtly repositioned as a resource and an advantage in her ability to care for a child. She refers to her isolation and her solitary state as somewhat facilitating her ability to care ("to have a child, you know, I could do that, it's just me"), and implies that if she had other obligations she'd have to split her time and energy among them, but as a single, elderly woman she is perfectly positioned to devote her attention to a foster child. Following on the heels of this reinterpretation of her vulnerability, Auntie Ma also frames her financial motivations quite candidly and matter-of-factly. Rather than shying away from her need, in both these circumstances, Auntie Ma makes her vulnerability a primary pillar of motivation in her willingness to foster Meili.

Meanwhile, middle-aged state orphanage and INGO employees frequently complained that no one but poor, elderly women would dare take in such "difficult" children. By their estimation, such needy alliances were understandable given both parties' social abandonment in modernity, but they were also disadvantageous because poor, elderly women were of "low quality," meaning they lacked the requisite education and culture to rear Chinese children poised for adoption to prominent Western nations. State orphanage and INGO monitors' prejudice toward poor, elderly women are reflective of government-sponsored discourse that emphasized the making of modern individuals into "high quality" citizens through education, enterprise, and development.[6] Given the perception of retirees as physically and socially marginal, orphanage and INGO workers were skeptical about whether such persons could be remade into "high quality" citizens and thus, subjected them to much scrutiny, surveillance, and critique.

For instance, middle-aged orphanage workers often speculated that elderly foster parents were primarily and problematically motivated by their poverty to foster disabled children. As one INGO director once scoffed, "Who would take in these 'cp kids' [kids with cerebral palsy] if not for the money?" The same employees who spent many hours caring for disabled children in the orphanage and monitoring foster placements often stammered under their breaths that they themselves couldn't imagine caring for or taking in "such difficult children." In this way, middle-aged orphanage workers perpetuated the belief that only those in truly desperate, or commensurate circumstances of social abandonment, would take in such highly undesirable children. Yet it was also such persons who were unfit to provide "high quality" care to orphans.

Furthermore, while orphanage workers imagined the child's care to be difficult, foster mothers often felt caring for a child was simple work. For example, one afternoon, out in the village of Daling, Mrs. Wang, the state orphanage foster care director, Huilan, a foster care monitor, and I visited a very elderly prospective pair of foster parents. When Mrs. Wang asked the couple whether they felt they could handle a disabled child from the orphanage, the old man responded with his eyes twinkling and raucous laughter, "Suibian! Suibian dai haizi!" The phrase, *suibian* and the response, roughly means something like, "No problem, whatever," or "It's easy to raise a child!" The old man's laughter and words visibly alarmed Mrs. Wang and Huilan, who shot back a whole host of questions and admonishments about how children from the orphanage with diseases were fragile and required constant care, and would certainly not be as easy as this couple expected. The old man and woman, however, did not seem dissuaded. On many occasions, I'd heard foster mothers similarly scoff, "Why, it's easy to raise a child. To feed and clothe a child? How hard is it?"

However, middle-aged orphanage monitors clearly bristled at this commentary, charging that elderly foster mothers did not take seriously the time, energy, and expenses it takes to raise a child. The monitors were also angry that foster mothers often misunderstood stipends meant for the children as wages or other compensation. Foster mothers, however, remarked frequently and proudly on their own frugality, because they believed it was an important skill in being a parent and raising a child. They felt that by making the money they were given stretch further and further each month, they were managing their resources with the utmost care and responsibility. They were proud of their ability to skimp and save in ways that distinguished them from the middle-aged orphanage and INGO women who monitored their caregiving.

Indeed, the middle-aged orphanage and INGO monitors, particularly Teacher Liu, the director of Mercy Care, and Huilan, the state orphanage foster care monitor, experienced stress in caring for their own biological families alongside their supervision of elderly foster mothers. As aforementioned they were often critical of these elderly women's financial motivations, but they themselves complained of the economic constraints on their own family lives. Teacher Liu once said to me, "It takes at least three people to raise a child; two just won't cut it!" She and Huilan relied on their parents and their in-laws to provide live-in care to their children while they worked long hours at their jobs. They often complained tearfully that raising children in modern China was arduous and draining, a stark contrast to the foster mothers' depictions of the relatively inexpensive, simple daily tasks requisite for child-rearing.

Even as middle-aged INGO and orphanage workers find foster mothers' vulnerability and poverty wanting, elderly foster mothers exhibit pride and security in their ability to provide care to foster children as solo parents on limited budgets. This is significant because despite their "low status" in the Chinese imaginary and their attested vulnerability in aforementioned scholarship, elderly foster mothers do not view themselves as victims of their social circumstances, nor do they behave as confined or constricted by their limited finances. Foster mothers reposition their social and economic vulnerability as a resource in their provision of good foster care and their work as good foster mothers.

In the next section, I demonstrate that through the bonds of fosterage that develop between elderly foster mothers and abandoned, disabled children, foster mothers experience certain economic, social, and political rehabilitation. I aim to show that this rehabilitation is perceived as a surprising affront to the very middle-aged INGO and orphanage workers who facilitate these fosterage placements, thickening this intergenerational ambivalence and foreshadowing a remarkable reversal of intergenerational influence.

Fosterage as Social Rehabilitation

Foster mothers cited many benefits from foster relationships that ranged from a boost in their own self-esteem to a raising of their status in the eyes of the community and even the state. Throughout my fieldwork, I observed that raising a child clearly gave these retirees a sense of purpose and heightened self-worth. Taking these children to the market or playground, or just out into the public courtyard gave isolated elderly an excuse to engage with their neighbors and their community. As foster parents developed pride and protective qualities over their children, they began to see themselves as valuable to community and society.

Hence, foster parents often proudly cited the work they were doing for these "pitiful children" as *gongxian*, or an act of civic sacrifice or duty. They felt that caring for a child, especially a child abandoned within the institutions of the state, recuperated their self-worth as active and important members of Chinese society. Most important, perhaps, the obligations created between children and foster parents reintegrated them into distinct social roles in family life, as they now became primary caregivers in family-like relationships. Although many of these children, especially because of their impairments, could not or would not be able to offer the foster parents much care now or in old age, the mirroring of the intergenerational contract in these relations, wherein these children and elders offered emotional comfort and solace to one another in the face of abandonment by their biological parents and children respectively, should not be overlooked (Croll 2006).

As poor, elderly women took on the role of foster mothers, they became visible and notable in their sacrifice not only for their foster children, but also for the Chinese state. In fact, their usage of the term "gongxian" to describe their motivations for fostering is highly significant in that gongxian is the same term that the Chinese government once employed to solicit the service of its people for the Communist Revolution and still uses to commend citizens for their sacrifices of extraordinary civic duty. Whether foster mothers were conscious of it or not, in suggesting that their kin work was a kind of gongxian, they appropriated the language of the Chinese state, suggesting that their service had distinct ties to the maintenance of political life and order.

This type of repositioning is noteworthy given the state's relative abandonment of poor, elderly women, as well as middle-aged orphanage and INGO care workers' criticism and discrimination toward elderly foster mothers. Because the state orphanage provided the infrastructure and funding for foster

care placements, they also conducted monthly visits to monitor the quality of
the foster mothers' care. Given the aforementioned suspicion of their motivations, as well as frequent criticism of their child-rearing and disciplinary methods, hygiene, and lack of education, foster mothers often resented these visits
and the surveillance of the state orphanage and INGO care workers. When I
accompanied such middle-aged employees on their monthly visits, foster parents were often carefully compliant toward state orphanage workers. However,
when I returned by myself, they confided in me that they begrudged the disre-
spect and subordination these employees conveyed. As one foster mother complained, "To them we are nothing more than *baomus* [a Chinese term for maid]."

Foster mothers also resented that they were left out of the loop in terms of
being told where and precisely when their foster children would be adopted.
When children were adopted, the orphanage policies demanded that any visits
between foster parents and adoptive families be conducted at the state orphanage or at a hotel. After adoptions, the orphanage also specified that any communication between adoptive families and foster families be conducted through
the orphanage. Orphanage officials stated that the reasons for these policies
were for the protection of the children and the adoptive families. They said
that they worried that foster families would try to solicit money from adoptive families, putting the state in an awkward position. But by concealing the
foster families' homes and lives from view, they also frustrated adoptive families who longed to have a relationship with their children's foster families. In
many cases, communication was nonexistent or strained. When I visited foster
mothers throughout China, they implored me to inquire about the whereabouts
of children adopted to places like Chicago or Atlanta, as they complained that
the orphanage never mailed their letters or provided them any communication from these adoptive families. They tearfully wondered what had become
of these children they raised, incredulous that adoptive families could be so
cruel as to cut off communication, and highly suspicious that it was the orphanage that was responsible for the lack of communication.

Although foster parents were clearly in a subordinate position with respect
to the authority of the state orphanage and INGO employees, their relationships with their foster children often compelled them to resist the power and
purview of the state. In March 2012, foster mothers in a rural foster care project
outside the capital city organized to demand higher wages from the municipal
orphanage that sponsored them. While at first glance such conflict may appear
to confirm foster mothers' self-interested or financially driven motives, foster
mothers in rural Daling were not merely lobbying for more money, but for the
privilege of taking in additional children. So motivated and compelled were they
by the needs of these children that each of them agreed to take on additional
third child, but they also demanded that compensation be raised. Because of a

significant shortage of foster mothers, the orphanage, which found itself in a superior position of monitoring these relationships, suddenly found themselves subordinate to the foster mothers' demands.

Many foster mothers, after falling into a deep depression after the adoption of a child, refused to take in another foster child from the orphanage. The orphanage, which relied on these mothers' care to alleviate its own financial burden and ready the children for international adoption, was placed in the desperate position of pleading with these mothers to take another child. In one instance, Auntie Lu, a foster mother who had fostered a child whose mother was incarcerated, ultimately persuaded the orphanage to let her keep the child into adulthood, despite the fact that children of the incarcerated are not technically eligible for state social welfare or adoption (Keyser 2009). Such instances demonstrate how foster mothers, motivated by their love and care for foster children, not only resist the state, but also gain substantial leverage over their circumstances due to these surprisingly empowering relations.

Despite the orphanage's complaints that Auntie Ma had been noncompliant with the orphanage staff and lacked discipline with her foster daughter, as Meili's adoption to the United States approached, orphanage workers began to encourage Auntie Ma to take in another child following Meili's departure. However, Auntie Ma provided multiple excuses: she didn't have any young children's clothes anymore, only clothes suitable for an older child, and she said she couldn't handle an older child at her age. Meili, her third foster child, would be her last. In so doing, Auntie Ma, like the other foster mothers before her, gained political leverage in that her important kin work becomes a service that the state covets.

Fosterage as Intergenerational Reversal

What my research shows is that despite their structural positions of relative power, middle-aged state orphanage and INGO workers are actually influenced by socially marginal foster mothers and their foster families. Throughout my fieldwork, I observed that despite the power middle-generation care workers held over foster mothers, they not only found themselves unable to control or reform these elderly women's behaviors, but were also influenced by their kin work and care. In other words, as I looked beneath the visible expressions of disgust and frustration on behalf of the middle-aged workers, I eventually saw through to a certain envy of their seniors that belied a deep insecurity and vulnerability in modern Chinese social life.

Even beyond the confines of these trying structural relationships, other middle-generation parents struggled to reconcile foster families' relative insecurity with the enviable emotional bonds they shared. One afternoon after I tutored Auntie Lu's foster daughter Pei Pei, her biological daughter Kaili, and Auntie Lu's sister-in-law's daughter in English, the sister-in-law, Mrs. Hu, accompanied me out to the curb. Thrusting a bottle of lotion into my hands, she thanked me for tutoring her daughter, remarking that she wished she had more to give me, but was grateful for the time I had spent with the girls. She bemoaned Auntie Lu's deplorable circumstances, particularly the fact that as a poor widow, she had no choice but to foster two children, in addition to her biological daughter, who suffered as a result. But then, tears began to fill her eyes as she reflected more. "But you see the way my daughter makes fun of me, of my Mandarin, the fact that she's rebellious and doesn't listen. Kaili [Auntie Lu's biological daughter] doesn't do that, certainly not Pei Pei [Auntie Lu's eldest foster daughter]. Auntie Lu may be poor but she's home all day with those girls. The three of them are so close, so they'd never mock her. My husband and I work long hours, so we're hardly there for our daughter. You see she's smart, but she doesn't respect us. What do you do with such rebelliousness?" she pleaded with me.

What was remarkable about this exchange were some of the underlying circumstances of insecurity in Auntie Lu's family that Mrs. Hu claimed to pity but ultimately overlooked because of the close bonds the foster family shared. Auntie Lu was a widow who relied on the stipends provided to care for her two foster daughters and some of the income of her eldest son to pay the family's expenses. Their household was one of the poorest I visited, with five people crammed into a two-bedroom apartment. Kaili, Auntie Lu's eldest biological daughter, was performing quite poorly in school, while Mrs. Hu's daughter was exceling. And yet it was Mrs. Hu who found herself tearful and distraught upon the curb that evening. She envied the closeness of Auntie Lu's family, the time she had to give to her children, and the respect that she saw conveyed between parents, children, and siblings. With her comments and her tears, Mrs. Hu intimated a state of fundamental insecurity faced by many young people in China, despite the relative stability of their social and economic circumstances.

Like Mrs. Hu, the middle-aged orphanage and INGO monitors, particularly Teacher Liu, the director of Mercy Care, and Huilan, the state orphanage foster care monitor, who were critical of elderly foster parents' modes of discipline, pitiable circumstances, and lack of education, were also anxious about their own trying relationships with their children and somewhat wistful about the foster mothers' close relationships with their foster children. When I left China in 2012, Huilan had just been promoted to director of foster care at the municipal orphanage, but the promotion left her with a certain ambivalence. In an e-mail written to me about her promotion, Huilan admitted that she struggled with feelings of inadequacy at doing this job of supervisory fosterage when she was such an absent parent. She realized that the new job would take her further away from her family, but in some ways it would also connect her with the lifestyle and values that she longed for from her childhood. Although she, like other middle-aged monitors, had once admitted to me that she could never care for such complicated children, she confided in me that she was moved by the sacrifices these women made. Throughout our time together, Huilan had often stressed that foster families had taught her that age was not a prerequisite to caring.

When one considers the demographic liminality of the so-called sandwich generation, those post-1980s Chinese only-children tasked with the nearly impossible responsibility of caring for their children and elders simultaneously, Huilan's insecurity and vulnerability is hardly surprising. And yet, relevant literature on shifting demographics in China too often stresses the vulnerability of the elderly over the insecurity of China's educated middle class. While Yan and others have argued that such insecurity tends toward rampant individualism and incivility, I detected a more subtle process of social change occurring among the generations in foster kin work in Guangxi, China.

Even though middle-aged, educated, middle-class women like Mrs. Hu, Teacher Liu, and Huilan harped on the insufficiencies of foster mothers and foster families, registering and scrutinizing their "low quality," they were nonetheless moved and affected by the close bonds that fosterage produced that they lacked in their own family lives. I suggest INGO and orphanage personnel criticized these poor, elderly women and the way they were raising their foster children because they found something in their own family lives wanting. The bonds of fosterage and the difficulty they presented to the Chinese state were interpreted as contestations precisely because of the social vulnerability of these youthful caregivers. If elderly foster mothers were truly marginal, expendable, "low quality" individuals, their actions would not have been so highly scrutinized and monitored by these state employees. Instead, their actions cut to the heart of shifts in the generational life of Chinese families, undermining middle-aged Chinese women's own normative notions of family, relationship, and success.

Elderly Foster Parents as Agents of Social Change

Although such conflictual relationships between elderly foster mothers and middle-aged care workers are perhaps not immediately recognizable as intergenerational contracts, I suggest they provide an important reinterpretation to previous studies of filial piety and intergenerational family life. Elementally concerned with future well-being, foster mothers and middle-aged care workers negotiate intergenerational relations of care along both nonbiological and biological lines. Traditional studies of filial piety in Asia have been relatively closed to less conventional relations like fosterage. What is striking is that in these nonbiological intergenerational relationships among elderly foster mothers, middle-aged care workers, and foster children, filial piety is reinterpreted in ways characteristic of biological intergenerational contracts. For instance, Croll (2006) argues that far from the intergenerational contract falling by the wayside, generations are taking new steps to invest in reciprocal relations of care as a strategy to combat the lack of support given to elders by Asian states. However, Croll, like others, emphasizes the ways in which elders are adjusting to ensure their old age security amid new patterns of family and production initiated by middle-aged youth. Hence, the argument about reinterpretation represents seniors' strategies toward generational security as a marked *response* to youthful change.

Whereas China's youth have often been characterized by their individualism, market-driven attitudes, and entrepreneurship, the elderly have been rendered fundamentally insecure. Yet, in the practice of foster care, we note that elders are actually far more proactive in combatting their own insecurity and adjusting to shifting patterns of family life in modernity than their youthful counterparts. Indeed, as Mrs. Hu, Teacher Liu, and Huilan bemoan the difficulty of their modern lives and wistfully and enviably observe the foster families, they are a composite picture of inaction, regret, and insecurity. I want to suggest that this reversal of roles demonstrates a defiance of demographic fates by savvy yet caring elders, whose commitment to transnational kin work and willingness to build relationships across biological lines speaks to their agency and adaptability. Far from merely responding to the world around them, seniors like Auntie Ma recognize that they are living in the best of times and make the most of new opportunities despite their social and economic insecurity. Meanwhile, China's youth seem remarkably paralyzed by their own burdens and insecurities, limited by their notions of family, relationship, and prosperity that are confined to neat, modern lines.

NOTES

1. All names are pseudonyms for the protection of informants.
2. Guangxi is an Autonomous Region located in southwest China.
3. Whereas residential patterns have shifted in many parts of China, my fieldwork demonstrates that brides still traditionally move in with their in-laws following marriage in Guangxi. This leaves families that are without sons particularly vulnerable and helps to explain the extremely skewed gender ratios in regions such as Guangxi.
4. For the way in which experiences during the Cultural Revolution produced fragmentation of the self and internal censorship which cause many individuals to keep silent about their suffering, see in particular, Kleinman et al.'s "Introduction" in *Deep China* (2011).

5. The 1950 Marriage Law stressed reciprocal obligations of parents and children for the welfare of the family. The 1980 Law, which replaced it, clarifies children's obligations to provide for their parents and gives parents the right to prosecute their children if they fail to do so. In collaboration with the 1980 Law, the *Jiating Shangyang Xieyi* (Family Support Agreement), a voluntary contract between parents and children, has been widely implemented throughout the countryside since 1985. As late as 2006, a government white paper entitled *Development of China's Aging Affairs* encourages parents and children to sign the *Jiating Shangyang Xieyi*. Most recently, in August 2012, China's National Bureau of Senior Affairs released the New 24 Filial Exemplars, which aim to protect the rights and interest of seniors by further conscripting their children in obligatory care. Hence, far from obsolete, the institution of filial piety is being notably reinvigorated by China's government, even as it is being reinterpreted by families and scholars of social life. For an excellent review of these recent developments and the place of filial piety in contemporary society, see Qi 2014.

6. This emphasis on high quality (*suzhi*) employed by the Chinese government in population campaigns to express that the goal of modernity is not only to decrease the population size, but also to improve the population quality has been widely studied (Anagnost 1997, 2004; Bakken 2000; Friedman 2006; Greenhalgh 2010; Jacka 2009; Murphy 2004; Sigley 2009; Wang 2010).

5

Negotiating Sacred Values

Dharma, Karma, and Migrant Hindu Women

MUSHIRA MOHSIN KHAN AND KAREN KOBAYASHI

In recent years, there has been a significant increase in the South Asian immigrant population as well as a concomitant rise in multigenerational South Asian households in Canada largely due to the sponsorship of older parents (Statistics Canada 2013).[1] Recent research suggests that immigrants are twice as likely to live in multigenerational households as compared to nonimmigrants (Battams 2013). Cheuk Fan Ng, Herbert Northcott, and Sharon Abu-Laban (2007), in their study on South Asian older adults living in Edmonton, Alberta, also found that compared to South Asians who had immigrated in early to midlife, those who had immigrated in later life were more likely to live with their adult children and/or spouse than alone. Indeed, India and Sri Lanka, with close to 5,185 landings between 2005 and 2010, top the list of source countries with the highest number of parent and grandparent sponsorships (Citizenship and Immigration Canada 2013).[2]

These two significant sociodemographic shifts have important implications for intergenerational support exchanges in South Asian immigrant families in Canada. In this chapter, we employ a life-course perspective to explore the feminization of kin work in immigrant families and the complexities inherent in intergenerational relationships within the diasporic South Asian community. We provide important cultural insights into evolving concepts of care and the negotiations, ambivalences, and contradictions that immigrant South Asian women experience in trying to sustain a moral, caring self and to maintain their interpersonal relationships.

Ten immigrant South Asian women revealed during in-depth interviews that their care of older adults was performed in the context of *dharma* (moral duty) and *karma* (fate) and their own obligations as people of particular social positions; there is, however, an inherent fluidity in these cultural values. Simply put, the values of dharma and karma are being redefined in this diasporic context. In this chapter, we discuss how the ideal of the dutiful daughter-in-law or the obedient daughter, and the kin work that is central to such identities, are being negotiated in Canada. We conclude with a discussion on how immigrant South Asian women may employ spirituality and religious beliefs as coping mechanisms to offset the unique challenges they encounter in the provision of care to older relatives.

Situating the Study

The feminization of kin work in immigrant families merits singular consideration given the inequalities that it perpetuates both within the family and outside of it. Usha George (1998, as cited in Spitzer et al. 2003), for example, has pointed out that kin work within South Asian families is highly gendered and deeply embedded in the very formation of women's "ethical and moral selves" (268). Similarly, in an ethnographic study on immigrant South Asian women in British Columbia, Sukhdev Grewal, Joan Bottporff, and Lynda Balneaves (2004) found that an important theme running through the interviews with female participants was a sense of duty and obligation toward the family, which the authors describe as the ideal of the South Asian woman as the dutiful wife, the obedient daughter-in-law, the nurturing mother, and the self-sacrificing caregiver.

The provision of care and support to older relatives (usually by daughters/daughters-in-law) has been linked to the Hindu concepts of *seva* (selfless service), dharma, and karma (Acharya and Northcott 2007; Sharma and Kemp 2011). Upholding the norm of filial piety espoused within these concepts can also be perceived as an indicator of a person's respect and appreciation for his/her culture of origin (Raffety, this volume). Specifically, Manju Acharya and Herbert Northcott (2007) observe that older Hindu grandmothers from nuclear and extended families living in Great Britain consider ethnic identity and tradition as important indicators of mental health. Older adults whose granddaughters had an exclusively Asian or Hindu identity and who embraced South Asian cultural values were more likely to be perceived as having better mental health in comparison with those whose granddaughters reported a British ethnic identity. Further, Sharon Koehn found that older immigrant South Asian women in her study tended to characterize the heightened independence of young women in Canada, and "the greater likelihood that they will work outside the home and prefer a nuclear family living arrangement," as selfish, robbing them "of the opportunity to be cared for in the way that they have provided care for their own elders" (2009, 591).

Emerging evidence from some urban centers in South Asian countries, however, suggests that women's growing economic independence brought about by higher education and sociocultural shifts has redefined the traditional mother-in-law/daughter-in-law power differential (see, for example, Masvie 2006; Vera-Sanso 1999). Indian mothers-in-law in Chennai (formerly known as Madras) who coreside with their daughters-in-law, for example, provide essential noneconomic support (childcare, and household chores such as cooking and cleaning) in lieu of a guarantee to be taken care of in old age (Vera-Sanso 1999). This raises three questions: (1) To what extent do important life-course transitions such as migration affect the nature of intergenerational family relationships and exchanges within diasporic South Asian households? (2) How do immigrant South Asian women negotiate the simultaneous challenges of settlement, kin work, and multigenerational coresidence in a new land? and (3) How are the cultural values of dharma and karma negotiated in a transnational context?

Theory and Methods

The Theoretical Toolbox

We use a life-course framework to provide insights into how immigrant South Asian women perceive their social world and negotiate the processes of migration and intergenerational family relationships. The life-course perspective takes into account the dynamic interaction of lived experience and sociohistorical context as well as the intermingling of subjective and shared meanings that shape lives over developmental and historical time (Cohler and Hostetler 2003). Such a perspective allows for the exploration of continuity and change in people's lives that is brought about by interpersonal, structural, and historical forces (Elder and Johnson 2002). Using this approach, we were able to trace the unique continuities as well as the vicissitudes that shaped the lives of the immigrant South Asian women in our study over time. It particularly helped us to establish links between the various stages in participants' life-course trajectories, such as their early life in the country of origin with mid-to later life experiences in Canada as immigrants and as caregivers within a transnational context.

Some basic concepts from the life-course perspective that were useful in our analysis included: "cohort," or a group of persons who were born during the same time period and who "experience particular social changes within a given culture in the same sequence and at the same age" (Hutchison 2010, 11); "transition," or a change in role or status; "trajectory," or a long-term pattern of continuity and change, which includes several transitions; "life event," a major incident or occurrence that may be sudden and abrupt and may have long-term ramifications; and "turning point," a life event or transition that results in significantly altering one's life-course trajectory.

Guillermina Jasso (2003) suggests that given the major changes associated with migration, immigration itself is an event that qualifies as a turning point. In this study, for example, immigration was a turning point in the lives of the participants that altered their sociocultural environment, familial relationships, and perceptions of the self, beliefs, and expectations. Similarly, the arrival of the participants' older relatives within a few years of their own migration to Canada was another "point of reckoning" (Evans et al. 2008, 7) that involved recognition of the complexities of coresidence and caregiving and their significant adaptation to their changed social circumstances.

The life-course perspective proved useful in acquiring deeper insights into the transnational spaces inhabited by the women in this study, and into the processes of identity construction and meaning making that they engaged in as they made sense of their lives as immigrants, mothers, daughters-in-law, partners, students, employees, and most importantly, as women of color in an unfamiliar land. In addition, it reflected the ways in which participants renegotiated their sense of place and identity relative to evolving social contexts, changing realities, environmental exigencies, and Westernized views of gender and culture, particularly in the provision of care to their older relatives.

Listening to their stories, we realized that the identities of these women were fluid and relational (West and Zimmerman 1987); the self was socially constructed and reconstructed in accordance with the circumstances they faced, building upon past memories, internalized moral and religious values, and "hopes and fears for the future" (Brunner 2003, 182, as cited in Heyse 2011, 201). The life-course perspective was thus useful in understanding the participants' embeddedness in multifaceted and dynamic intergenerational and conjugal relationships. Indeed, as Neena Chappell and Margaret Penning note, "We are all embedded within social environments; we live our lives interacting with others in multiple and often overlapping contexts" (2009, 111).

Data Collection

We used purposive sampling methods to recruit ten adult female participants who had immigrated to Canada from South Asia within the past ten years as either Economic or Family Class immigrants, who were citizens or permanent residents, and who coresided with their older relatives at home. Refugees and temporary foreign workers were excluded in order to maintain relative sample homogeneity. One participant, Seema (pseudonym),[3] was selected despite the fact that she did not currently coreside with her older relatives because her husband's parents, who had lived with her for four years, had recently returned to

India permanently. The rationale for interviewing her was based on two important considerations: (1) when she contacted the researchers, Seema appeared very keen on sharing her experiences; and (2) the researchers believed that Seema's past lived experiences of coresidence with older relatives would provide unique insights into the sociocultural and structural factors that may contribute to a breakdown of the sponsorship relationship.

Site of Recruitment

With regard to the recruitment site, Shyam Grover has noted that not only does the Hindu temple satisfy the important function of fulfilling the religious needs of the immigrant South Asian community, it also acts as a site for socialization and the reproduction of the "rich cultural heritage" (1978, 14) of South Asia. Contact information for members of the planning committee of the local Hindu temple was obtained from its website. These individuals are all volunteers who are primarily involved in organizing cultural and social events within the community and are not a part of the religious order of priests and the clergy. E-mails were sent out to eleven such individuals, informing them about the purpose and nature of this study. A letter of invitation containing details about the study and the researchers' contact information was also appended to the emails, requesting members to either forward it to recently landed South Asian immigrant women via e-mail or to inform them by word of mouth. These members, therefore, acted as broadcasters who facilitated access to the population of interest.

As Table 5.1 indicates, of the ten recruited participants, eight women were originally from India and two were from Sri Lanka. All participants were university educated and between thirty-two and forty-five years of age. Several held a bachelor's degree or higher from an institution in their country of origin. All participants were raised in an urban setting, and belonged to upper middle-class families.

All participants were married, fluent in English, and had been engaged in paid employment in their home country prior to marriage. All were presently engaged in paid employment in the receiving country, that is, Canada. Seven participants had at least one child, and three had no children. Seven participants currently coresided with their parents-in-law, two coresided with their parents, and one participant had coresided with her in-laws in the past. The older relatives of the participants were between sixty-two and seventy-nine years of age.

Qualitative Interviews

Ten semistructured, face-to-face, open-ended interviews were conducted between September and December 2013 at locations chosen by the participants. The interviews, which lasted approximately two to three hours each, were

TABLE 5.1

Profile of Study Participants

Participant's name	Country of origin	Age of participant	Education	Lives with parents-in-law	Lives with parent	Has children	Engaged in paid employment in Canada
Anshu	India	35	Bachelor's degree	Yes		Yes	Yes
Joyita	India	35	Master's degree	Yes		Yes	Yes
Aarti	India	40	Bachelor's degree	Yes		Yes	Yes
Smriti	India	40	Bachelor's degree	Yes		Yes	Yes
Chandana	Sri Lanka	44	Master's degree		Yes	Yes	Yes
Sudha	Sri Lanka	32	Bachelor's degree		Yes	No	Yes
Seema	India	37	Master's degree	*		Yes	Yes
Khushi	India	33	Bachelor's degree	Yes		No	Yes
Priya	India	32	Bachelor's degree	Yes		No	Yes
Gayatri	India	45	Bachelor's degree	Yes		Yes	Yes

* Lived with parents-in-law in the past.

conducted primarily in English. Jennifer Yusun Kang (2012) has pointed out that unique challenges regarding interpretation and communication may arise in interview situations where the two languages being used are typologically different (for example, Korean and English). In this regard, the first author's ability to converse in and understand several South Asian dialects helped in establishing rapport with participants. For example, some participants used the word *desi* (local/Brown) to describe diasporic South Asians, and *gore log* (White people) to describe mainstream (mainly Caucasian) Canadians—terms the first author was familiar with given her identity as an immigrant South Asian woman.

Also, although the sample was not limited to university-educated women, all the participants who contacted the researchers were highly educated professional women from South Asia. The fact that these women approached us voluntarily indicates that this study may have been perceived as an opportunity for participants to voice the unique challenges that they faced in the context of resettlement, multigenerational living, and in the provision of care to their older relatives. Finally, the choice of the Hindu temple as a site for recruitment implied that all participants would identify as Hindu; this ensured sample homogeneity in terms of religious affiliation and allowed us the latitude to compare and contrast the narratives of the participants within a specific religious context.

The data collected from the interviews were analyzed following Jane Ritchie and Jane Lewis's analytical hierarchy method, which involves building findings from raw data (2003, 217). In interpreting the findings from this study, however, the following limitations must be taken into consideration. First, this research was limited to a purposive sample of only ten South Asian women who core-side with their older relatives in Canada. The participants in this study were not randomly recruited, and, therefore, are not necessarily representative of the South Asian immigrant population in Canada. However, as Yvonna Lincoln and Egon Guba (1985) have pointed out, this trade-off affords the researcher the advantages of acquiring deep and detailed understandings of social processes (Cuadrez and Uttal 1999). Further, we invited participants to share the stories of their lives with us; the in-depth nature of their narratives (each interview lasted approximately two to three hours) offers nuanced insights into the experiences of this group of immigrant South Asian female caregivers. Despite the relatively small sample size, the interviews themselves were information rich (Baker and Edwards 2012), and we stopped collecting data once theoretical saturation had been achieved, that is, when no new or relevant insights seemed to be emerging from the data (Bryman 2001).

Second, this research would have benefited from interviews with both members of the dyad, that is, with the members of both generations, to understand better the unique challenges of multigenerational living. Future research should look into the dynamics of intergenerational relations that have been highlighted in this study, for example, the evolving mother-in-law/daughter-in-law relationships in diasporic South Asian communities over time.

Finally, the sample was not limited to participants with children in order to increase the sample size. Past research has suggested that for adults who are simultaneously providing support to dependent children and aging parents, the provision of care may be viewed as both a joy and a burden due to the element of reciprocity attached to coresidence (Igarashi et al. 2013). Although this study includes some participants with children, it would be worthwhile to explore the lived experiences of the so-called sandwich generation in order to acquire deeper insights into the unique challenges that middle-generation South Asian immigrants may face in the process of care provision and in the negotiation of familial bonds, as Neda Deneva in this volume has done.

Results

The findings indicate that for the participants in this study, the challenges of settlement as immigrants were exacerbated by the complex and dynamic interplay of multigenerational living, their early-to-mid-life socialization in their country of origin, and adherence to culturally prescribed, gendered rules of conduct.

In this section, we discuss: (1) how the Hindu philosophical framework of dharma (moral duty) and karma (fate) was viewed by the participants in fluid and relational terms resulting in a constant negotiation of the culturally ascribed identities of "the dutiful daughter-in-law" and "the obedient daughter" in a transnational context; and (2) women's agency, structural constraints, and the complex subtleties of multigenerational living and support exchanges in South Asian immigrant households. We conclude with a discussion on the implications of these findings for policy and practice.

Hinduism as a Way of Life: Dharma, Karma, and Migrant Hindu Women

Glen H. Elder (1998) has suggested that individuals move through a sequence of age-graded events, settings, and social roles that are structured by social institutions; these societal forces define normative pathways that provide templates or road maps for individual lives (Crockett 2002). The family cycle, with its focus on role sequences related to marriage, to childbearing, to early parenthood, to "launching and settling" the child, to the empty-nest syndrome, and to grandparenthood, is an example of how the family as a social institution defines paths or trajectories comprising sequential statuses and the transitions between them (Crockett 2002). In Hinduism, the life course of the individual is divided into four distinct stages or ashrams: in the first stage, *brahmacharya*, one is a celibate student; in the second stage, *grahastya*, one is bound by household duties; in the third stage, *vaanprasthya*, bonds to worldly affairs are loosened; and finally, in the fourth and final stage, *sannyasa*, one is free from material concerns and seeks spiritual fulfillment (Choudhry 2001).

The women in this study had all been kin-scripted, or conscribed to age and gender-related kin work that was structured by cultural and religious scripts about family roles (see Deneva, this volume). Thus, their sense of identity centered on being the dutiful wife, the obedient daughter-in-law/daughter, and the loving mother. All participants had been married between the ages of twenty-one and twenty-seven, through traditionally arranged endogamous (within the same caste and/or clan) alliances. The courtship period, if there was one, was brief and quickly led to the wedding. After the wedding, all participants moved in with their husband's family. These women embraced the culturally prescribed role of the dutiful daughter-in-law with enthusiasm by taking on the responsibility for domestic chores such as cooking, cleaning, performing *poojas* (prayers), and providing childcare to the young children (not necessarily their own) in the household. As one participant, Smriti, described: "First I was a student, a daughter, and then I became a daughter-in-law and a wife. There is a time for everything. It has all been written down before your birth." The internalization of the normative family cycle and the timing of lives was also evident post-migration in the participants' decision to co-reside with their older relatives in Canada. It was clear that there was an underlying notion of reciprocity, a repayment of debt, and an abiding sense of gratitude toward their older relatives. As Joyita stated: "Look, my father-in-law has worked very, very hard to bring up my husband and his brother. . . . There was never any question about where they [her husband's parents] would live after retirement. If we lived in India, they would live with us, if we live in Canada, they will live with us. This is our time to repay their debt."

Previous research has also suggested that early-life experiences in the country of origin are often overlooked as an important marker in the simultaneous reproduction of inequities in the immigrant experience (Heyse 2011; Weerasinghe and Numer 2011). For the women in this study, their sense of self and identity, both as immigrants and in the context of their relationships with their older relatives, were couched in the religious and moral values that they had been socialized to take up during their early lives in South Asia. Despite their Western education and the exposure to modern values of egalitarianism and notions of free will, these women displayed a deep appreciation for South Asian values, particularly the Hindu philosophical concepts of dharma and karma, the sacramental aspect of marriage, respect for older adults, and their social duty toward the family and community.

The life-course perspective also recognizes that life-course pathways of individuals are embedded both within sociocultural as well as historical contexts, culminating in the production of cohort effects, that is, the sharing of distinct formative experiences at the same point in the life course (Hutchison 2010). Swarna Weerasinghe and Matthew Numer (2011), for example, found that the physical, emotional, and social health and the leisure activities of immigrant South Asian widows in Canada were significantly influenced by childhood behaviors and their early lives in their countries of origin. For the women in this study, adolescence in an urban, metropolitan context in South Asia resulted in the creation of a cosmopolitan identity, particularly with regard to education and career goals; specifically, all participants admitted that they were encouraged to cultivate personal ambition and drive during their adolescent years by their older relatives.

Given this inordinate focus on personal ambition and academic success, it was paradoxical that eight of the ten women quit their respective jobs in the country of origin once they got married. Collectively, their response as to why they transitioned out of the labor force was because they felt this was the dharma of a married woman. They had been socialized to believe that, as per the Hindu code of conduct, their primary duty was to respect the wishes of their new family. Their mothers or other female members of their family had instructed them to focus on "winning the hearts" of their husband's family, particularly during the crucial early days of their marriage. The following statement by Aarti provides insight into how internalized cultural values shaped notions of selfhood, interpersonal relationships and kin work among these women:

> You know, in our culture, mothers whisper into their daughter's ear at the *bidai* [Hindu bridal send-off ceremony] that sasuraal mein theek se rehna, sabko kush rakhna [behave yourself in your husband's home and keep everyone happy]. This is how we lived our lives back home, and this is how we live our lives here [in Canada]. Always caring for others [laughs].

Dharma, or moral duty, then, was an all-encompassing theme, inextricably woven into the narratives of all participants: according to them, it was their dharma to obey their parents and marry a life partner chosen by the elders of the family; it was their dharma to quit paid employment and look after the needs of their husband's family in their country of origin; and it was their dharma to peacefully coreside with, and provide care to their older relatives in the host country. Pittu Langauni has pointed out that among the patrilineal communities of South Asia, it is also the dharma of Hindu parents to see their daughter happily married off and after the wedding ceremony, "like a snake casting of [sic] its skin" (2005, 90), the Hindu bride is expected to bury her past and start her life with a new identity that is ascribed to her by her husband's family. It is her moral duty, therefore, to sustain and nourish her new family by effortlessly adapting to her new role as wife and daughter-in-law, and failure to do so invites social disapproval and dishonor. This internalization of cultural values acted as a coping mechanism for the participants in this study as they simultaneously negotiated the challenges of settlement and kin work.

To illustrate this point: upon immigration, the women in this study discovered that they had to reenter the workforce in order to financially support their families, resulting in significant role conflict and distress. On the one hand, they were duty bound to provide care for the members of their family inside the home, and on the other, they had to face the challenges of a fast-paced and competitive professional world outside the home. Although their reentry into the labor force brought about feelings of empowerment, having to work at low-paying jobs despite their high professional credentials in order to acquire Canadian work experience resulted in a situation fraught with uncertainty and feelings of powerlessness. Given this perceived disruption in their family and work trajectories, however, these women expanded their definition of dharma to incorporate the provision of financial security to the family. Education and paid employment, despite being incommensurate with their academic and professional credentials, was regarded as a means to further the economic development and advancement of the family and not as a way to establish their personal autonomy and independence.

And, as testimony to culturally scripted and enduring family roles, although migration had resulted in a new openness in communication, respect for each other's space, and a more egalitarian view of marriage as far as spousal relations were concerned, the contribution of these women toward the maintenance of their families, and their labor, both outside as well as inside the home, went largely unrecognized. As Geeta Somjee explains: "The Hindu woman has a very definite self-respect, but it stems from her identification of 'self' with 'family'" (1989, 34). So pervasive is this internalized concept of moral duty, that for the participants in this study, it was difficult to outline their caregiving practices quantitatively. Care was inextricably intertwined with spirituality and religious beliefs, and tending to the physical, material, and emotional needs of their older relatives was perceived as an act of reciprocity or a (re)payment of debt to aging parents—the duty of all devoted offspring. As Sudha maintained, "I don't measure my care." Also, all participants felt that living with their older relatives was a good deed that would eventually be rewarded. As Joyita explained: "See, in Hinduism, there is this idea of karma [fate]. Whatever you do comes back to you in this life. So if I have kids, they will also take care of me."

A Tricky Negotiation of Sacred Values

Upholding the sacred values of dharma and karma and engaging in culturally prescribed kin work also proved challenging for many participants in the context of migration. Most admitted that they often felt overwhelmed by having to constantly juggle the diverse needs of their children and those of their older relatives. Chandana's father, for example, liked to listen to the radio all day, and since he was slightly hard of hearing, he turned up the volume in order to be able to listen. The noise from the radio, however, proved distracting for her children, especially when they were trying to study for tests. Similarly, like the adult children of older migrants in Parin Dossa's essay (this volume), the participants in our study faced a similar dilemma around dividing familial time between the previous and future generations. Anshu described how she found it stressful and difficult to reorganize her schedule on days when she had to drive her in-laws to the local Hindu temple or to medical appointments, and also take her children to their after-school extracurricular activities.

With regard to long-term and end-of-life care, when participants were asked about the provision of instrumental care to their frail older relatives when the need arose, most emphatically stated that they would quit their jobs and stay at home to look after their older relatives. In what was a paradoxical theme then, many participants stated that they felt "really scared" about the future. Most admitted that it would be easier if they received culturally appropriate support services at home. Although the actual provision of care, such as assistance with activities of daily living (ADL), did not appear to be an issue, many participants agreed that they would welcome support for the caregiver.

Thus, for the women in our study the values of dharma and karma were being renegotiated in the diasporic context. But despite the desire to conform to the culturally prescribed ideal of the dutiful daughter/daughter-in-law, optimal care for older relatives was often compromised by a singular lack of awareness of available support services, reliance on informal sources such as the larger South Asian community for information, their financial insecurity, and the challenges of settlement.

Agency, Ambivalence, and the Complex Dynamics of Multigenerational Living

The life-course perspective recognizes that individuals participate in the construction of their lives through the exercise of human agency, or the use of personal power to achieve their goals (Hutchison 2010). Although the women we interviewed were constrained to a large extent by culturally prescribed norms and values as well as their historical circumstances, they nevertheless exercised personal agency in directing the course of their lives. When her husband's parents arrived in Canada, for example, Anshu unequivocally laid down certain ground rules: "This is my house, and if I didn't tell them [her in-laws] the rules on Day 1, I felt like I would lose all control." She set up a self-sufficient room with kitchen and bath for her in-laws on the lower level of her house separate from the other bedrooms on the upper level, thus ensuring that her in-laws were comfortable, while at the same time, maintaining her own need for privacy and personal space.

Similarly, during the initial days of their arrival in Canada, Aarti's in-laws would often accompany her family on restaurant visits. The following excerpt from Aarti's interview demonstrates how immigrant South Asian women use creative solutions to overcome some of the challenges associated with coresidence and care provision to older relatives:

> This whole eating out thing became very painful. We had a family ritual, right, that once a month, we will go to a nice Canadian restaurant, and just relax. My in-laws, when they moved here, also used to come with us. But there were so many problems. They are completely vegetarian, so we always ordered veggie stuff. But that was also a problem. They would say that "Okay, this is veggie, but they must have used this oil to fry beef, so we cannot eat this." So, when this happened four-five times, the children were getting very frustrated, so I said, "You know what, you stay at home because I will not disappoint the children for that." Now we go out, just the four of us, and my in-laws, they stay at home.

Technology was also used as an effective means of negotiating the unique challenges accompanying care provision to older relatives. Gayatri, for example, discovered that long-distance calls and the accompanying telephone charges had increased significantly ever since her husband's parents moved to Canada. This presented her with a difficult conundrum—on the one hand, she did not want to sound disrespectful by asking her in-laws to stop making calls to their friends and relatives in India, but on the other, she did not like the idea of paying exorbitant telephone bills. She was eventually able to resolve the issue by purchasing a tablet for her father-in-law, thereby enabling him to make Skype calls to his relatives back in India. This anecdote also underscores how technology may play a crucial role in maintaining social networks in the country of origin for individuals in diasporic communities.

The participants in this study also reached out to the local South Asian community, which served as an important source of social support for them. When Seema's father-in-law suffered a stroke, for example, a South Asian friend stepped in to take care of her children. Additionally, both Seema and her friend took turns delivering their home-cooked food to her father-in-law who would not eat the food served at the hospital for religious reasons. The larger South Asian community also served as an important informal source of information, both with regard to the challenges associated with resettlement as well as the support services available for older adults. A family friend who had immigrated to Canada thirty years ago, for example, provided Anshu with details about the volunteer services available for older adults in the municipality in which she lived.

The findings from this study also indicate that perceptions around privacy and personal space differed based on socioeconomic, cultural, and individual factors. For a few participants, their dharma dictated that they ensure the well-being of their older relatives to the utmost, even at the cost of sacrificing their own comfort. For example, Anshu's family sold their home and bought a considerably more expensive house in a South Asian neighborhood when her parents-in-law moved to Canada. Anshu's former house had too many stairs, which her arthritic mother-in-law would not be able to negotiate, and her father-in-law would be able to socialize with other older adults of his age in the area. An unfortunate consequence of this, however, was that Anshu had to take up an evening job in order to offset the increased monthly mortgage payments, which had placed her family under significant economic strain.

On the contrary, the notion of privacy and personal space was not an issue for those women who coresided with their own parents, to the extent that the close physical proximity of their parents fostered a sense of safety and security based upon a lifelong relationship of faith and trust. These findings indicate that the dynamics of multigenerational living, particularly with regard to decisions around privacy and personal space in diasporic South Asian households, may be subjectively experienced and negotiated.

Further, coresidence with older relatives was regarded as beneficial for the transmission and maintenance of cultural values. Past research (e.g., Spitzer et al. 2003) has suggested that within immigrant families, women typically shoulder the responsibility of inculcating and fostering cultural values in their offspring. The women we interviewed revealed that their inability to successfully juggle the demands of the workplace with their caregiving duties meant that they passed on this additional responsibility of cultural transmission to their older relatives. Like the grandmothers in Dossa's essay (this volume), the older relatives, usually the mothers or mothers-in-law, of the women we interviewed took it upon themselves to teach cultural values to their grandchildren. Additionally, they provided essential support at home, particularly with regard to childcare, cooking, and cleaning. Ho Hon Leung and Lynn MacDonald (2007) have highlighted the benefits of multigenerational living in their study on immigrant Chinese women in Toronto. "Caregiving and care receiving experiences," state the authors, "can involve a high level of reciprocity, particularly if the elderly parents are able and healthy" (2007, 19).

Janice Keefe and Pamela Fancey (2002) have also pointed out that the caregiving literature tends to focus more on the care provided to older adults than on the support older adults provide to their families (also see Zhou, this volume). In fact, contrary to Sharon Koehn's (2009) observations on the intricate and delicate complexities of the mother-in-law/daughter-in-law relationship within immigrant families, the findings from this study indicate that there was a strong element of reciprocity, protectiveness, and affection attached to this relationship—while the mothers-in-law assisted with childcare and other domestic chores (particularly the care of the "difficult" father-in-law), the daughters-in-law provided essential emotional support to them, at times even standing up for their mothers-in-law in domestic arguments. Smriti, who works as a laboratory assistant in Canada, respects and appreciates her mother-in-law for helping out with childcare and cooking: "She is like my best friend. I come home from work, and we both sit down with a cup of tea. I tell her each and every thing that happened that day, and she tells me about my father-in-law's latest *tamasha* [fuss] [laughs]." This feeling of solidarity could be attributed to their exposure to Westernized ideals of feminism and the emancipation of women.

Although their relationship with their mothers-in-law was by and large harmonious, for the women in this study, it was their precarious relationship with their fathers-in-law that warrants attention. Although the internalized values of dharma, karma, and respect for elders precluded them from getting involved in open arguments with their older male relatives, deep feelings of resentment at outright displays of patriarchy simmered within the participants. As Thomas Blair (2012) has also pointed out, these demonstrations of patriarchy could be attributed to the fact that from the perspective of the fathers-in-law, migration to Canada may have resulted in a loss of role and status within the family, particularly in the context of having to depend on their daughters-in-law for their essential needs.

Therefore, although their internalized cultural and religious values may act as a coping mechanism for urban, highly educated immigrant South Asian women, their globalized and transnational identities may produce ambivalence and uncertainty with regard to their sense of self, and may result in a complex (re)negotiation of interpersonal relationships and kin work.

Agency and Structural Constraints

A key reason offered by the participants for their choice of Canada over for example, the United States as the receiving country, was the assumption that Canada had far friendlier policies with regard to the sponsorship of older relatives, and their subsequent care and support, in comparison to other immigrant-receiving countries. Both factors are particularly salient and require our careful consideration. Indeed, as these women encountered the harsh realities of settlement and changing sponsorship policies, and as they experienced marginalization, discrimination, and downward mobility, they often found themselves questioning their decision to leave behind their comfortable lives in their country of origin. Learning through their transnational networks about the "successful" lives of their peers in South Asia, particularly with regard to the pursuit of Western lifestyles and extended networks of social support, often led to feelings of regret and ambivalence among participants.

The example of Seema, whose parents-in-law returned to India permanently to provide in-home care for her father-in-law because of insurmountable financial and physical constraints, highlights the dilemma of reconciling the ideals of filial obligation, love for one's parents/in-laws, and dharma or moral duty with structural constraints, such as lack of culturally appropriate support services, their visible minority status, complex re-credentialization processes, and low socioeconomic status. Indeed, these factors may act as barriers to the provision of appropriate care for older relatives. The complexities of intergenerational relationships, along with broader structural factors such as lack of culturally congruent care, therefore, may result in the termination of a multigenerational living arrangement. This finding provides support for Laura Funk and Karen Kobayashi's (2009) argument that filial care work needs to be understood contextually as involving family and relationship dynamics, as well as broader, macrolevel factors at the social, political, economic, and cultural levels.

In sum, despite their exercise of personal agency, for the contemporary urban, middle-class women in this study, financial insecurity, disruption in their normative life-course trajectories, underemployment, lack of access to relevant information, the physical and economic burden of care provision to older relatives, and the complexities of multigenerational living, combined to produce conditions of multiple jeopardy.

Implications and Recommendations

As an immigrant-receiving country with a below-replacement fertility rate, Canada needs university-educated and highly skilled immigrants to contribute to the growth of its economy. Canada's points system of immigration, which favors highly qualified applicants, has done fairly well in attracting university-educated immigrants since the 1970s up until the early 2000s; however, more recently, the poor economic outcomes of well-educated new immigrants with regard to the relative wage gap and other challenges of settlement are indicators that the country has actually fared poorly in comparison to the United States (Statistics Canada 2011). These challenges, as Yanqiu Rachel Zhou (this volume) has also pointed out, are further exacerbated for many immigrant South Asian women who must simultaneously juggle the demands of settlement with the challenges of providing care for their older relatives at home. Although their older (mainly female) relatives may provide support at home, such as assistance with childcare and domestic chores, previous research has indicated that mul-tigenerational living is reciprocal and beneficial only when older relatives are healthy and able (Leung and McDonald 2007).

The findings from this study also suggest that these women may employ spirituality, religious beliefs, and dharma and karma as coping mechanisms to offset the unique challenges they encounter. In fact, as Saba Mahmood (2011), in her ethnographic study of women's piety movements in the mosques of Cairo, Egypt, has pointed out, cultural and historical factors often mediate the sense of self and agency. For the women in her study, it was not necessarily freedom from the traditional patriarchal structures that they sought; rather, they used those very cultural prescriptions to navigate the dynamic terrains of settlement and kin work, developing a fluid and relational sense of self in the process. Indeed, to quote Mahmood: "What may appear to be a case of deplorable passivity and docility from a progressivist point of view, may actually be a form of agency—but one that can be understood only from within the discourses and structures of subordination that create the conditions of its enactment" (2011, 14–15).

Given this, from a Westernized perspective on freedom and equality, there is also a strong possibility that the stoicism and resilience of these women may render their needs invisible in the broader domain of policy and practice. For example, some of the tasks categorized as "elder care" on the 2007 General Social Survey (GSS) include meal preparation, house cleaning, laundry, sew-ing, and assistance with personal care such as bathing (Statistics Canada 2008). This quantification of care work may lead to misleading statistics for immigrant South Asian caregivers as they may conceptualize the provision of care to their older relatives in more culturally congruent, fluid and less structured terms. The implications of this incongruence in the understanding of what constitutes care work may be that immigrant women remain unaware of available programs and services and therefore experience caregiver burden in multiple domains, including finances and health, as they try to do everything themselves.

In addition, of those who were aware of existing resources, most indicated that given the lack of culturally appropriate support services in their region, they would quit the paid workforce to provide care to their older relatives should the need arise. This attitude is problematic on three levels: (1) It would result in a significant loss to the Canadian economy; (2) It would hinder the advancement and economic development of their families, further perpetuat-ing the cycle of disadvantage; and (3) Loss of income may not even be an option for those women who may be severely socioeconomically disadvantaged in the first place, possibly leading to a breakdown of the sponsorship relationship. It is of vital importance, then, to recognize that although internalized cultural val-ues may guide the caregiving decisions of immigrant South Asian women, it is often not cultural factors, but rather, more pragmatic structural issues such as lack of or an inability to access relevant information and support services, that may create conditions of multiple jeopardy and disadvantage among recently landed South Asian caregivers.

This finding underscores the need to develop channels of information dissemination that are specifically tailored to the needs of this vulnerable group. For example, the local Hindu temple could act as a site for educational seminars, particularly with regard to the availability and utilization of services, and training skills in role management, resource planning, and time management (Gupta and Pillai 2002). Similarly, as one participant in this study suggested, the local recreation/community center, by holding periodic South Asian seniors' socials, could serve as a cost-effective initiative for the informal dissemination of information, as well as a means to meeting the social needs of South Asian older adults.

As a way of fully appreciating the unique challenges that recently immigrated South Asian caregivers face, this study makes an important contribution by contextualizing their migration and caregiving experiences based upon biographical, historical, structural, and cultural factors. For example, as is the case in contemporary China (Raffety, this volume), modernization and urbanization have led to the rise of the nuclear family in South Asia, culminating in an erosion of the extensive social support networks of the past (Allendorf 2013). These factors may have ripple effects in diasporic communities in that they may increase the likelihood that South Asian immigrant parents will coreside with their children, requiring an increase in the sponsorship of older parents under the Family Class category. Further, with longer life expectancies, older adults are likely to cohabit with or continue to be dependent on their children for extended periods of time, leading to an increase in the physical, emotional, and economic responsibilities placed on the younger generation (Gulati and Rajan 1999; Zhou, this volume). As Barbara Gee and Ellen Mitchell (2003) have predicted, multi-generational living in Canada will continue to rise, thereby providing increased opportunities for daily contact and social interaction among family members, be those good or bad (Mitchell 2007).

NOTES

1. Parts of this chapter have been derived from the first author's unpublished master's thesis.
2. The United Nations Statistics Division (2012) defines South Asia as a geographic region comprising nine countries from the Indian subcontinent: Afghanistan, Bangladesh, Bhutan, India, Iran, Maldives, Nepal, Pakistan, and Sri Lanka.
3. We have used pseudonyms for all participants to preserve anonymity and confidentiality.

6

Transformations in Transnational Aging

A Century of Caring among Italians in Australia

LORETTA BALDASSAR

There is a growing body of research on the role of Information and Communication Technologies (ICTs) in transnational family life. While much of this literature examines the challenges of distance and the negative impact that the absence of kin has on family relationships, there is also a tendency to assume (or assert) that ICTs nevertheless have revolutionized our capacity to care across distance and are transforming forms of caring in the process. My own contributions focus on transnational aged care and propose that this polymedia environment is facilitating caregiving through the creation of new forms of "being there" or copresence across distance (Baldassar 2016). However, with some important exceptions (e.g., Madianou and Miller 2012), few publications, my own included, provide detailed evidence of *how* the changes in communication technologies have transformed the ability of transnational families to be copresent, above and beyond the fluid mobility patterns described by Neda Deneva (this volume). In this chapter, I attempt to chart these changes and transformations over time, using the century-long history of Italian migration to Australia. I compare and contrast the forms of caregiving, kin work, and copresence experienced by four cohorts of Italian migrants in relation to specific time periods. These time periods are characterized by distinct and diverse access to various communication technologies that facilitate different methods, modes, and meanings of distant care.

The chapter begins with a brief overview of the history of Italian migration to Australia and a summation of the methods of my research. I then define what I mean by transnational aged care, explain how people use communication technologies to care for each other across distance, and make the case that keeping in touch and copresence across distance is a form of care. Each cohort is then discussed in turn, drawing on fine-grained ethnographic longitudinal data, to examine how communication technologies are used to deliver a sense of "being there" for migrants and their aging parents across distance. I argue that these practices and processes of copresence across distance are forms of caregiving and kin work that deliver the emotional and moral support that is constitutive of family relationships (see Yarris, this volume). The aim of this chapter is to assess if and how ICTs have transformed processes and practices of caregiving and kin work across distance, including delivering new forms of copresence. I argue that different forms of copresence are created in each cohort. In particular, recent polymedia environments facilitate synchronous forms of copresence that are substantively different from earlier asynchronous forms. In the concluding section, I discuss the contributions and limitations of polymedia environments and their role in transforming the practices and processes of caring, kin work and copresence across distance.

One Hundred Years of Italian Migration to Australia

Italian labor migration to Australia represents the final chapter in the massive Italian diaspora that saw over twenty-five million people depart the peninsula between 1861 and 1965. More than half of these migrants were headed for neighboring European countries like Germany and Switzerland. The remainder sought their fortunes in far more distant destinations, mainly the Americas but also Africa. Just under 1 percent of these emigrants made it to Australia and, for the purposes of this chapter, are divided into four main cohorts: a relatively small but foundational prewar (1900–1940s) cohort; the largest and most substantial cohort of postwar (1950–1960s) arrivals; a smaller post-1970s (1970–1990s) cluster; and a recent new migration (post-2000). This trajectory means that Australia has a relatively young Italian immigrant population, although most first-generation migrants from the postwar period are now over sixty-five years of age, and there is a vibrant second and growing third generation.

There are several key characteristics that help to contextualize transnational care in Italian-Australian migration history. Italian emigrant departures of the first two cohorts did not represent an even spread across the peninsular, with the majority hailing from the southern regions as well as the Veneto and Lombardy in the north. They were all leaving for largely the same reasons and with similar motivations. They were "worker-peasant" (Holmes 1989) and labor migrants escaping extreme poverty, a crippled economy, and limited job prospects (Isastia 1991, 236). Most, however, intended to repatriate once they had raised enough money to "set themselves up" (*sistermarsi*) in their hometowns, an intention supported by repatriation statistics. For example, between 1960 and 1969 a staggering 71 percent of arrivals from the Veneto region returned.

The proportion of Sicilian immigrants returning to Italy was 19.7 percent and of Calabrians, 14 percent (Thompson 1980, 231).[1] Thus, for most Italians, their migration project is best understood as a family economic strategy undertaken to facilitate an eventual repatriation. This meant that the actions, hopes, aspirations, and imagination of these migrants were oriented homeward. In many ways, their migration project, and the act of migration itself, was an expression of family caring, copresence and kin work. Both migrants and their stay-behind kin were engaged in the joint project of family betterment and *sistemazione* (establishment) and in this way could be said to inhabit shared transnational life worlds, social fields, and imaginaries, as noted by Kristin Yarris (this volume) in relation to grandmothers taking care of grandchildren.

In this chapter, I take a migration cohort approach to aging because the comparison of various cohorts lends itself to an analysis of life-course transformations as well as the changes in the migration process over time. Furthermore, because these migrations are best understood as a family economic strategy, in particular those of the pre- and postwar, caring is defined in broad terms such that caring for the elderly was just one part of caring for extended family as a whole. The prewar migrants arrived as young adults and most grew old in Australia, only able to participate in the aging of their parents from afar by providing much needed remittances. The postwar migrants had a similar trajectory, though with relatively high rates of repatriation and even higher rates of return visits, which permitted them a closer involvement in their parents' aging. The post-1970s migrants and the recent arrivals, as well as their homeland kin, enjoy very transnational lives, aging together across distance. Although each cohort experienced family separation and absence, family members were very much copresent in each other's lives despite the distance. However, as shall be shown, exactly how this copresence was experienced and enacted changed considerably over time with the development of new communication technologies.

Distant Aged Care

The definition and forms of family caregiving that have featured in my analysis to date (Baldassar 2007, 2008; Baldassar, Baldock, and Wilding 2007, 2014) are drawn from Janet Finch and Jennifer Mason's (1993) classic five types of family care. However, for the purposes of this chapter I reorganize these into three types of care. I combine emotional/moral support and practical care (giving advice and sharing information), because these forms of care can most obviously be delivered across distance. I also combine accommodation (providing a place to live) and personal care (hands-on caring, including feeding and bathing), because these two forms of care would appear to require physical copresence. I retain financial care as a distinct form, which I define primarily as remittances, as these are the traditional mainstay of the migration process (see Mullings, this volume). Elsewhere, I have theorized these types of care as delivering different forms of copresence across distance (Baldassar 2008, 2016a)—including physical, virtual, imagined, proxy, and simultaneous—and I compare these across the various migration cohorts.

All four migration cohorts show evidence of the same three patterns of reciprocal care: routine, ritual, and crisis. Routine patterns of care are distinguished by their regularity. Although the method and mode of this form of care has changed significantly over time, this pattern of distant care represents the bulk of the time-intensive kin work of emotional and practical care that forms the mainstay of transnational family relationships (see Coe, this volume; Yarris, this volume). For example, the more assiduous family members of the early cohorts, usually daughters and their mothers, exchanged careful and detailed monthly letters full of expressions of love and advice. An essential part of this early pattern of routine care included the sending of regular remittances: both financial, which Supriya Singh, Anuja Cabraal, and Shanthi Robertson define as the "currency of care" (2010, 249); and social, which Peggy Levitt defines as including "ideas, behaviors, identities, and social capital" (1998, 926). Today, routine distant care is still largely about emotional and practical care, but is more likely to take the form of daily SMS messages and Facebook posts, as well as weekly phone or Skype calls, often involving multiple family members. Ritual patterns of distant care, which also flow both ways—between migrants and homeland kin—are characterised by emotional and moral support, but also often include significant and costly gifts, including large sums of money, jewelry, household goods, or financial contributions toward a car or house. This pattern of care has remained surprisingly constant, represented by the exchange of cards and gifts for special anniversaries and birthdays. However, in the more recent cohorts, the direction of the flow of gifts has changed. Whereas earlier migrants sent gifts home, recent migrants are more likely to be recipients of gifts. Crisis patterns of care have also remained constant across the cohorts. These comprise responses to moments of emergency—including illness, death, and dying—and are characterized by increased communication using all the modes available. Today, crisis care often involves family members visiting each other for lengthy periods to provide personal care.

Arguably, all these forms (practical, accommodation, financial) and patterns (routine, ritual, crisis) of care are expressions of emotional and moral support. It is difficult to argue that emotional/moral support is less necessary than other forms of care, and that it is not in itself a type of care, particularly in transnational contexts where there are limited opportunities for other forms of caregiving (Baldassar and Merla 2014). This form of caregiving is particularly evident, and often in an enhanced form, at times of crisis, particularly when deaths in the family occur (see Dossa, this volume). Further, distant care often involves the coordination and delegation of care by others, which we might call caring by proxy. Majella Kilkey and Laura Merla (2014) argue that it is important to acknowledge that a family member who delegates caregiving to a third person or institution does not automatically step out of circuits of care but may still be "caring about" the person (Fisher and Tronto 1990, 40), stay informed of the level and quality of care provided and be ready to step in when needed. Mirca Madianou and Daniel Miller (2012) have shown how intensive this form of caring by proxy can be, particularly for migrant mothers of stay-behind children. Caring by proxy raises the issue of the care and kin-work duties left to those who do not migrate (see Yarris, this volume). As has been noted, Italian migration was part of a family economic strategy to provide the finances to sustain the family back home, who in turn cared for the young and elderly in the migrant's stead. I return to these issues in the final section of the chapter and discuss the limitations of distant care.

Methodology

Most of my three decades of ethnographic research has focused on the postwar migrants (mainly from the Veneto and Sicily) and comprises participant observation and oral history interviews with dozens of families in both Italy and Australia.[2] Data were collected in several extended fieldwork trips in 1987–1989, 1993, and 1999–2000 with families primarily in Perth, but also in Queensland as well as their kin in Italy (Baldassar 2001). This research involved extensive participant observation and follow-up over time with approximately twenty families, including over forty formal in-depth interviews focused on postwar migrants and their Australian-born children. In a later, second project I also conducted research on the post-1970s cohort, which involved approximately twenty families and includes over forty interviews with migrants, their Australian-born children, and their kin living in various regions throughout Italy. This data forms part of a much larger collaborative study from 2000 to 2004 that focused on transnational family and caregiving relationships comprising over 200 ethnographic interviews and participant observation with Australian migrants and their parents living in Ireland, Italy, the Netherlands, Singapore, and New Zealand, as well as refugees from Iraq and Afghanistan and their kin living in transit in Iran (Baldassar, Baldock, and Wilding 2007). My research on this topic is ongoing, and I have since conducted further research as well as follow-up interviews (Baldassar and Merla 2014).

A third project, conducted from 2005 to 2009, involved the collection of approximately 170 life history interviews and 4 group discussions (in which 115 individuals took part) with postwar migrants from across Western Australia (see Iuliano 2010). More recently, from 2010 to 2012, I conducted research that included the cohort of new arrivals in Perth and Melbourne. This project examined economic, political, sociocultural, and kinship ties to homeland and included a survey comprising over 600 respondents and a series of focus group interviews conducted with a range of representatives from each of these major migration cohorts (Baldassar and Pyke 2014). Research on the prewar migrant experience is scantier and thus I draw on my own personal Italian migration history as well as the available literature, in particular Jaqueline Templeton's (2003) precious study of letters written by early Piedmontese migrants and their kin back home.

Pre–World War II (1900s–1940s) Cohort: Scripted Presences through Longed-for Letters, Sporadic Parcels, and Return Migration

The earliest arrivals from Italy to Australia began during the 1850s after journeys by ship that lasted three to four months. The first important technological change to impact transnational migrant relations occurred in the late 1860s with the introduction of steamships that significantly reduced the journey between the two countries to about five to six weeks. In this period, the largest single source of Italian immigrants was the northern region of Lombardy and, in particular, the central Valtellina in the province of Sondrio. Nearly two-thirds of Australia's Italian immigrants before 1900 hailed from Sondrio province, and almost half of all Italian immigration was from Valtellina alone (Templeton 2003, 14–15). Between the wars, most arrivals still intended to return, but the majority ended up staying for good. According to Templeton, "settled communities had developed in the 1920s and the idea of permanent settlement was beginning to take hold. . . . In almost every year between 1930 and 1937, women and children, often on prepaid fares, far outnumbered adult men" (2003, 29). These departures were family reunions; even the men migrating were the kinsmen of earlier migrants.

Detailed data about transnational care practices for the aged is hard to find for the prewar group. I have several interviews with descendants, but mostly my research folders comprise reflections about them by the postwar group. A common theme, evident in the quote below, is that the 1920s migrants "forgot their *patria*" or homeland. This impression was no doubt created by the long absences that were common for this group of migrants.

> Franco Zamin arrived in Australia just before the war and the manner in which he describes his past, clearly reveals the perceived differences between the two groups of migrants [pre- and postwar]. By the time he arrived, the 1920s group had decided to stay in Australia, they had "called

out" their wives and families and, as some would have it, had begun to forget their patria. Franco Zamin talks about himself as an "escapee," taking on the 1950s migrants' perceived attitudes of the early [1920s] migrants. He admits that for a time he forgot about Italy and concentrated on making a new life for himself in Perth. During one interview, in which both Franco and his wife were present, Franco waited for Maria to leave the room while she went to prepare some refreshments, before confiding in me a part of his past which he was not proud of: "I had forgotten my mother, I want to be honest, I had actually forgotten my mother. That's why she wrote to me via the Red Cross during the war. I should have written . . . but I got a car here, straight away. Of Italy? Who thought of them over there? I had forgotten my mother and everything."
(Excerpt from Baldassar 2001, 191)

Despite Franco's experience, the incidence of chain migration and marriage by proxy suggests that these migrants continued to be oriented toward their hometowns, although their ability to be in touch was vastly curtailed by lack of means. Several other interviews mention the prohibitive cost of postage stamps: "The story [Dad] always told was that for years the only money he spent was on stamps to write to mum and myself. He said it cost him one pound eighty. I'll always remember that amount" (Baldassar 2001, 210). One nonmigrant who stayed behind in the hometown recalled his delight as a child when the "rare" parcel arrived from "*la giù*" (down there, i.e., Australia). What is important to note is that the arrivals of the postwar group reinvigorated and reinforced the prewar group's connections to both hometown and patria.

Evidence that the 1920s migrants had not forgotten their patria, or at least, had not done so indefinitely, is provided by their trail of letters and repatriation and return-visit history. Most return visits only began in the 1960s when air travel became relatively affordable. Templeton's (2003) book of letters from the Valtellina provides evidence of significant letter exchange and travel between the two places. Templeton confirms that "returnees' tales and migrants' letters were important because they familiarized the idea of Australia. . . . As sojourners, they wrote of what to them was most important, commenting on work opportunities, or the lack of them, and the pay" (21–22). But mostly, writes Templeton, "The letters reflect the writers' preoccupation with their families, their financial or property interests that those families are managing, and friends and neighbors" (51). Key themes included frustration at the distance and not being kept properly informed: "I want to know how much there still is in the bank and what the countryside looks like and tell my son Vincenzo to write proper letters and to let me know all the family news as you don't tell me enough and even if you don't get a letter from me write all the same saying what you need and what's happening" (52). There were also frequent expressions of torment at not being appreciated or understood, as is evident in one man's account after eight years in the Australian bush:

> I got the letter from our Maddalena in which she tells me that you're all well. This was a great comfort for me and the rest of the letter was a great torment as she told me to come home so that we could all be poor together. Things seem to be very bad but I don't believe you are suffering from lack of food and drink and as for having to work too hard or being a bit short of money[,] that I can believe a bit and because of the war and it's the same here in Australia. Anyway, the war will end. . . . I'm sending you 10 lire because the job has come to a stop and I can't do without everything. (Templeton 2003, 58)

Templeton's detailed study of letters to some extent challenges the argument that letters were mostly formulaic, a thesis made famous by William Isaac Thomas and Florian Znaniecki ([1918] 1996). In their classic work, these authors argue that "Letter writing is for [the Polish peasant] a social duty of a ceremonial character, and the traditional, fixed form of peasant letters is a sign of their social function" (25). Categorized by the authors as a "bowing letter," "its function is to manifest the persistence of familial solidarity in spite of separation" (25), in which elements may be schematized (see also Stanley 2010). This said, the evidence provided above does support the argument of Madianou and Miller (2012) that these prepolymedia times were characterized by asynchronous communication and ritualized patterns of letter exchange that were more likely to provide limited impressions of distant kin rather than clear knowledge about the actual person. I return to these points in the analysis section at the end of this chapter.

Postwar (1950s–1960s) Cohort: Proxy Presences through Migration Chains, Regular Remittances, and Special Transnational Objects

The most significant cohort of settlers was, without a doubt, the postwar group, who arrived in the decades immediately following World War II. Even here, the conventional historical record suggests that the choice of Australia as a destination was, in many cases, largely due to the immigration restrictions in place in North America. The Australian nation was initially very reluctant to accept Italian immigrants given its White Australia policy[3] and trade union fears of competition from cheap labor. Some historians argue that it was pressure from the British and US governments, as well from the Vatican secretary of state, that led to the Immigration Agreement of 1951, which effectively facilitated the mass migration of Italians to Australia (Bosworth 1988). And yet, the letters in

Templeton's collection provide abundant evidence that the information provided by migrants and returnees was extremely influential in determining migratory routes, far more than any formal government policies.

It was not until the postwar period that access to phone lines became commonplace, although they were not necessarily ubiquitous in people's homes. As evident in the quote below, making a call may have involved a very public process. "In those days when we wanted to telephone his mother, we would have to phone the local bar down the street from their house. Someone at the bar would have to run up to the house and call them. Then they'd run down to the bar and we would call back. There was no such thing as a private phone call! The whole bar and most of the village participated in it somehow" (2001 project interview).

Although phone calls and landlines became more affordable and commonplace, they were still mostly used in routine or ritual patterns for special occasions. Letters and cards were still largely the mainstay form of contact, but by now postage stamps were easily affordable and parcels could be sent more often. We found quite a degree of variability in the frequency of letter writing and exchange, although a strong gendered pattern of women doing most of this form of kin work (di Leonardo 1987). Visits were also becoming more common. There were also many examples of special transnational objects including photos, *bonboniere* (keepsakes from weddings and christenings), and gifts that crisscrossed the ocean (Baldassar 2008, 257). Federica's experience is probably reflective of the norm:

> Federica and her family have generally maintained close and regular contact, although there have been what Federica describes as "dark periods" when she did not feel as emotionally supported as she wished: "I've felt that[,] well, I might as well be dead for them because you know, I'm so far away." The sense of isolation was exacerbated by contact being primarily by letter and infrequent phone calls, which gave Federica an unsatisfying level of detail about daily events; "I want to know exactly what's happening and like during the visit home, I used to find out that this happened . . . that happened, and I was reproaching my dad for not telling me, also the negative things like somebody died." These dark periods diminished as phone calls became more affordable: "At first it was really expensive so . . . you couldn't say much . . . But then when the price reduced—that was very, very important I think because, I mean[,] you can pick up the phone more or less any time and . . . check how things are going when . . . something worries you." (Excerpt from Baldassar, Wilding, and Baldock 2007, 209)

Most of the postwar arrivals were young adults whose parents could be classified as young-old enjoying a relatively high degree of independence.

Remittances continued to be sent home, particularly by those migrants who intended to repatriate. This money was often invested in new or renovated housing for the migrant and his elderly parents. As family reunion was the main migration policy, age was far less a barrier to entry than it is under the present points system. But it was also the period when migrants began to focus on settling in Australia. As certain parts of Italy began to enjoy an economic "miracle," remittances started to peter out and financial investments were directed toward Australia. Perhaps even more frequent than the exchange of phone calls in this period was possibly the flow of arrivals along migrant chains defined by kin and hometown networks. Elsewhere I argue that the visitor is a kind of proxy for the stay-behind kin (Baldassar 2008). Thus, these arrivals were a parade of proxy presences bringing news and gifts from home and in many ways embodying the longed-for faraway kin. The arrival of a townsman or woman or, especially, a sibling was like having a part of the homeland arrive.

In terms of aged care, what is striking about this period is not just the number of visits made by migrants to their homelands to see their elderly parents, but also the occasional rare and extremely celebrated visit by an elderly parent to Australia. I remember the visit of my paternal grandmother in 1969 very well. She spoke no English and made the long trip alone. She arrived at the start of summer and was aghast at my bare-footed existence, chiding me gently in a language I barely understood. By the end of the summer she could be found, shoes in hand, walking around the back lawn; she needed her shoes close by in case someone arrived and she had to put them back on quickly. I also remember my parents' deep disappointment that she had to return to Italy earlier than planned because a daughter-in-law was suffering a difficult pregnancy and needed her help. My parents often complained that we had her with us for just a few weeks in all her lifetime and their kin back home had her all the time. This complaint speaks to the tensions between migrants and their stay-behind relations about who deserved a mother's care. Were the postwar migrants who had decided not to repatriate as worthy as the stay-behind kin? By this time, migrants had ceased sending remittances, preferring instead to invest in their new homes in Australia. Inheritance rights reflect this social change with migrants often surrendering their rights to stay-behind kin in recompense for the aged care those relatives provided in the migrants' stead (Baldassar 2001).

Post-1970s Cohort: Virtual Presence
through Routine Phone Calls and Rare Visits

The post-1970s arrivals were not necessarily connected by chain migration links to the earlier cohorts. Many were skilled migrants looking for career prospects as well as those who had fallen in love with a traveling Australian. These arrivals often found employment within the Italian community as language teachers, welfare and community officers, and so on. The post-1970s period is characterized by more affordable and reliable landline phone calls, the exchange of cassette tapes, photographs, and even homemade videos, and increasing visits. While phone calls were becoming increasingly regular, providing access to more of the intimate details of everyday life, interview transcripts from or about this period contain a strong theme of frustration about trying to have a meaningful phone conversation without being distracted by the exorbitant costs. As one young female migrant exclaimed: "You can hardly concentrate on the call because you are worrying about how much it is going to cost." One informant described receiving motivational cassette tapes prepared by her sister to support her through a difficult divorce. This mode of communication is redundant now as the same sisters enjoy regular Skype and Face-Time calls today. But when the cost of phone calls was so prohibitive, the cassette tapes provided access to her sister's emotional support whenever it was needed (see Baldassar 2007).

The post-1970s cohort has perhaps been the quickest to take up new technologies in their transnational care practices, largely because they are the group with the most care obligations to elderly parents. Of all my informants, the case of Nina is perhaps the most poignant and representative (Baldassar 2007, 394–397). She left Italy to marry her Australian fiancé, largely against the wishes of her family, who felt it a weak justification to move so far away. I have argued elsewhere that the absence of an economic motive often resulted in migrants, particularly women, not being given what I term "license to leave." As a result, there were often tensions in the long-distance relationship whereby migrants felt they could not complain about their difficult experiences, because they were warned not to go in the first place. Nina suffered a burden of guilt for leaving her parents, compounded when her father died suddenly and she was unable to visit him in time. She dreaded that she would also fail to be with her mother on her deathbed. Nina visited as often as she could afford, at least every two years in the past decade. For her and her mother, polymedia arrived too late. Nina took the dramatic step of deciding not to visit anymore because leaving her mother was too painful for both women. On their first Skype meeting, Nina's mother was overcome with emotion and insisted the video be turned off because she could not embrace her daughter and seeing her was too painful a reminder of the distance.

New Millennium: Continuous
Copresence through Polymedia Potentialities

In recent years, there has been a new and significant cohort of immigrants with numbers matching those of the postwar era. These new arrivals are of a very different kind of migrant, although, like their historical counterparts of the postwar era, they are mostly young adults looking for economic opportunities and job prospects. Unlike their forebears, however, they are mostly well educated with good English skills and aspire to find careers in the professions and white-collar occupations. Arguably, the most important difference is their visa status. While the post-1950s cohort was encouraged to settle and stay in Australia, these recent arrivals are on temporary visas and are unlikely to be able to stay longer than a few years. Furthermore, the latter are more likely to be recipients of financial support from their families back home rather than providers of remittances (Baldassar and Pyke 2014).

While most of the postwar group have lost their parents, the recent migrants tend to have parents who are still young-old and relatively independent (Field and Minkler 1988). Today, the practice of transnational aged care is arguably increasingly becoming the same for all groups. How to care for aging parents, particularly the old-old, is a cause for concern for many post-1970s migrants today. In many respects, all groups approach transnational caregiving in much the same way, although there are some important differences, mostly to do with the so-called growing technological generational gap. It is to these contemporary practices and processes of distant aged care to which I now turn.

Distant Aged Care Today

The option of bringing elderly parents to live in Australia today is accessible to very few. The parent migration stream is extremely limited and costly, although growing. Parent migrants are people who enter Australia on Parent Visas (Subclasses 804, 838, 864). Applicants for these visas must be over sixty-five years. In just one decade, Parent Visa holders have grown from 513 people in the 2002 to 2003 Family Stream Migration to 8,725 in 2012 to 2013. The noncontributory parent category accounted for 27.9 percent of the family-stream pipeline of applications in 2012 to 2013 (DIAC 2013). Not all countries have equal access to visiting visas and those considered high risk of overstaying may not be issued a visa at all. There are also strict rules governing how long a visitor can stay in Australia and what level of insurance they must travel with. Elsewhere I have written about the lack of a transnational social policy that would govern the health and well-being of elderly visitors who, due to strict visa time limits, can be forced to depart the country despite being gravely ill (Baldassar 2014).

The more common practices and processes of contemporary transnational aged care comprise routine Skype calls, regular phone calls, and frequent text messages and e-mails reflective of the polymedia environment available to most middle-class migrants and their families back home today. Andrea's case, described below, represents a common pattern of transnational aged care today. Andrea is studying in Australia and his parents are young-old and quite independent. Even so, his mother Anna is a very attentive long-distance presence in Andrea's daily life. Anna sends Andrea texts every day; "even too often" bemoans Andrea. "She's always sending these stickers on Viber. They're kind of silly, but for her they are a way to tell me that she is thinking of me and that she is caring about me." Andrea feels he has to reciprocate by sending stickers back to his mother, but he has "trained her to accept that one or two a day is enough." Andrea says that he has had to become "religious" about "the weekend Skype call": "You have to have a really good reason to skip the call, like, you are dead." During the call, his mother and father both participate, but it is usually his mother who stays on the call the longest. "Dad will come and take a good look at me, see if I look okay and say 'Hi.' Mum will ask me lots of questions, go into detail: 'What am I eating? How am I sleeping? What am I feeling?' You know, she really worries about me and tries to look after me. . . . Of course, I like to see them too, but really once a week is even too much for me. It is an obligation."

Andrea will also exchange e-mails with his mother and some of his extended family, including his cousin who is about his age, and his close friends. He maintains a Facebook page and checks the pages of his friends and family both in Italy and in Australia. He feels he has a "pretty good idea" of how everyone close to him is "getting on" and that he wouldn't necessarily know any more if he were living in Italy. What is interesting about Andrea's experience is the sense of exasperation with how constant and intrusive communication with his family and friends in Italy is, particularly with his parents. This complaint is the opposite of the pre- and postwar migrants who bemoaned the scarcity of communication and its lack of detail. In Andrea's case, distance is no longer an impediment to the exchange of detailed knowledge about daily life in the way it clearly was for the prewar letter writers in Templeton's volume.

Although virtual forms of copresence are increasing, as people age, physical copresence in the form of visiting becomes less possible, specifically for the old-old. This said, the young-old are also enjoying new roles facilitated by new technologies and cheaper mobility, for example, the so-called flying grandmother, who is flown over to look after grandchildren for extended periods while parents have travel commitments of their own. A major impediment can be the generational divide in convincing elderly kin to take up new technologies, which often results in younger generations and a wider network of kin being co-opted into circuits of transnational caregiving to provide the technology that supports the long-distance care exchange. Unlike Andrea, a young single man with young-old parents, Alberto is middle aged with an old-old parent in Italy.

Every day during his lunch break at around 1 p.m., Alberto, who lives in Perth, Australia, phones his eighty-five-year-old father Angelo who lives in Rome, Italy. Angelo, who is not in the best of health, is usually sitting at the kitchen table having his morning coffee and bread roll. "It'll only be 6 a.m. in Italy, but Dad will always be waiting for my call," Alberto explains. Since Alberto's mother's sudden and unexpected death a year ago, Alberto, an only child, has tried to manage his father's increasing care needs from a distance. He took six weeks' unpaid leave from work to travel to Italy to arrange the funeral for his mother and put in place care supports for his father. Both Alberto and Angelo see aged care facilities as a last resort option; they are expensive and have a social stigma that reflects badly on families. Angelo wishes to remain living in his own home for as long as he can. Moving to Australia is not an option because of Angelo's failing health; furthermore, aged migration to Australia is costly with prohibitive requirements. Given the aged care regimes in both countries, father and son adopted the commonest solution and hired a domestic worker, Maria, to work from nine to five each day, preparing lunch and dinner, doing the cleaning and shopping and taking Alberto to his medical visits. Maria has agreed to move into the spare room as a live-in carer if Angelo's health deteriorates. A long-time family friend, Nadia, the daughter of Angelo's old friend and neighbor Nello, sets up a Skype call every Sunday when she visits her father who lives next door. Alberto feels this is the best way to "get a thorough update." Nello has a live-in carer who is also on hand at nights if an emergency arises. Alberto plans to spend all his recreation leave in Italy, putting some financial strain on his family in Perth, but fortunately his wife is supportive. Alberto's daughter Alana is planning to visit her grandfather while on an exchange student trip to Europe later in the year. (Excerpt from Baldassar et al. 2014, 156)

In contrast to Andrea, Alberto has quite a struggle to keep in touch with his father. Although the routine he has developed works adequately, he must rely on other people to facilitate the use of communication technologies.

New Forms of Copresence: Comparisons of Distant Aged Care across the Cohorts

Each cohort shows evidence of the same three patterns of care: routine, ritual, and crisis. For the prewar cohort, routine, and ritual care were delivered through letters and for many, over time, routine became ritual as letters decreased and became limited to ritual calendars of birthdays and anniversaries. Part of the pattern of routine care was sending regular remittances as well as entrusting a fellow migrant with news and cash to deliver to kin on their return. Importantly, the exchange of letters was often the kin work of certain actors: in particular wives, mothers, and sisters. Crisis care is evidenced in calling on the support of the Red Cross to find a kinsman who had fallen out of touch, and sending additional cash in hard times and additional (perhaps longer) letters with special news.

The postwar cohort, by the 1950s and 1960s, had access to telephones, at least for crisis care moments, but increasingly for ritual patterns of care to mark special occasions. On these occasions, more kin were conscripted into the kin work with the phone being passed around to more voices. Letters continued to form the mainstay of routine and ritual care but with more regularity, and usually between the same letter writers who formed the funnels of information, gathering and distributing to and from their networks beyond. The 1980s marked the beginning of the technological communication revolution, which affected the postwar and later cohorts. These technological advancements cut across social-class differences. Ritual care continued to be provided by letters and, increasingly, greeting cards. More dates were added to the ritual kin care calendar, including not just aging parents' birthdays and anniversaries, but also those of extended kin, including nieces, nephews, and cousins. Routine care became regular Sunday phone calls in which the whole family participated; letters as a form of routine care started to decline. Crisis care often took the form of a visit and/or an increase in all forms of communication with more regular phone calls and letters.

Since the 2000s, letters have virtually ceased. Telephone calls have become routine for all, particularly the elderly, and have become as well the ritual markers of distant care. Interestingly, crisis care is sometimes evidenced by the special use of the letter, which is nowadays a rarity. For example, sharing of seriously bad news—like major illness—may be shared in a letter as a way of marking out the specialness of the communication against the more routine forms. Visits have now become part of ritual care to mark the special occasions of the life course like birth, death, and marriage. For the wealthy, visits have become a feature of routine care, becoming annual or biennial. Most importantly, more kin are conscripted into kin work as younger family members are asked to assist the elderly with the new communication technologies. The new technologies of distant care are also transforming the gendered practices of kin work, as men become increasingly involved in managing the technologies including setting up the Skype call, downloading phone Apps, and maintaining the Internet hardware. In this way, circuits of care networks are expanding as kin who were not normally part of kin work become routine carers. In summary, families tend to utilize all the modes of communication available to them to exchange distant care.

While new technologies have reinforced the three main patterns of care described above in each cohort, they have also facilitated new forms of copresence across distance. Physical copresence remains the gold standard for all cohorts, achieved either through visits home or repatriations, and they are particularly important in periods of crisis care. For the prewar cohort, repatriation and a sistemazione back home was the ideal marker of a successful migration project. For the later cohorts, and all who decided to settle in Australia long term, the visit not only provides opportunities for direct hands-on kin work and care, but reinforces and reinvigorates family ties more generally. According to John Urry, these "intermittent periods of co-presence . . . are essential for developing those relations of trust that persist during often lengthy periods of distance and even solitude" (2003, 163).

Virtual forms of copresence are transforming the methods, modes, and meanings of kin work and distant care. The literature on the migrant letters exchanged by the prewar cohort describes these early missives as formulaic and standardized, performing a ritualistic social function of confirmation of family solidarity and duty (Thomas and Znaniecki [1918] 1996, 25). Remember, too, that many of these migrants would have had limited literacy skills. Madianou and Miller (2012) describe the key limitation of letters (and the cassette tapes that accompanied them when they became available) as "their lack of interactivity and simultaneity," which had the effect of exacerbating "inequalities and asymmetries" in the existing relationships. "The time lag between sending and receiving these communications also partly explains how communication often ended up becoming a more formalized or ritual exchange that was as much an expression of cultural obligation as it was of personal feelings" (Madianou and Miller 2012, 67). In contrast, the plethora of communication technologies available today for the aging postwar and more recent cohorts deliver forms of virtual copresence across distance that were not available before. This sense of being there across distance is not only provided by the content of the messages exchanged, but also by the very act—or kin work and care work—of creating the messages. Madianou and Miller describe the acts of communication in and of themselves, both the content and the form, as representing the phatic function of communication exchange in providing "an emotional reminder of the distant significant other" (75). Hence, the musical "ping" of a text message arriving as well as what it says are both perceived by the receiver as expressions of care and copresence.

It is this phatic function of communication exchange, along with the relatively unlimited access to a variety of modes of communication that characterise polymedia environments that together deliver new forms of copresence. Mirca Madianou highlights the capacity of new media today to deliver what she calls a form of "ambient co-presence" (2016, 183). For example, video-over-Internet platforms like Skype and FaceTime (where callers can see and hear each other in real time) allow groups of people to share a kind of constant connectivity, which for many delivers a sense of constant copresence; as if your family is always nearby. Elsewhere, I have described its key characteristics as being "live or real time," "streaming," and "immediate" (Baldassar 2016a, 153). In contrast to streaming copresence, texting by SMS or Apps like Viber and WhatsApp creates a form of copresence that could be defined as "intermediate" and "selective or discretionary" (153), because individuals choose when they will read and reply to messages. A feature of these text-based communication platforms is their storage capacity. Several informants mentioned the benefit of being able to reread messages (particularly useful when clarifying details about illness) and return to photos whenever they liked, something that can be done on mobile devices at any time and in any place. Although this form of copresence does not deliver the sense of "being there all together in the moment" that streaming or immediate copresence does, it can provide a strong sense that kin and friends are "there for you." In some ways this form of copresence is also a kind of ambient copresence, or continuous copresence, an ever-present, fully encapsulating sense of being there always in the background.

Conclusion

It is abundantly clear that there are differences in the regularity, frequency, and modes of care exchange between the various migration cohorts. Although all cohorts shared a similar set of patterns of care, the manner in which this care was exchanged and how often varies greatly. Furthermore, a major factor that impacts the experience of caring, copresence, and kin work appears to be dependent on the ability to experience and be experienced as actual persons, rather than either some ideal role type or a vague impression (see Madianou and Miller 2012). The time spent apart and the ability to experience moments of physical copresence in the form of visits is critical in this regard. Migrants in the prewar cohort could become increasingly unfamiliar to distant kin the more time they were apart. Their primary mode of communication—letters—did not easily counteract this process and could in fact compound it, with distant kin becoming relatively vague and impressionistic, creating "a kind of vicarious alternative to the actual person" (Madianou and Miller 2012, 148). In contrast, migrants who enjoy conditions of polymedia are able to share their actual selves with distant kin in real time, challenging the distinction between physical and virtual copresence (Madianou and Miller 2012).

A key difference in the type of copresence possible in the different cohorts is whether there is access to synchronous or asynchronous forms of communication. The emotional transnational imaginary that characterised the prewar cohort and asynchronous prepolymedia contexts were constituted by the shared family project of migration and were sustained by the exchange of letters, the sending of remittances, and rare but longed-for visits and repatriations. The form of copresence created in these contexts were mostly imagined and risked becoming attenuated, as migrants and their distant loved ones relied on modes of exchange that, over time, tended to deliver increasingly vague and impressionistic experiences of each other, although copresence could always be open to revitalization. Transnational aged care in this scenario mostly took the form of caring by proxy, in which the kin work of personal care was delegated to those family members who stayed behind and was supported by remittances, which represented and embodied the migrants' care. In stark contrast, the transnational imaginary that characterises distant family relations today is constituted by polymedia environments that facilitate synchronous copresence in which a form of self that more closely approximates the actual self can be exchanged, along with the possibility of a continuous feeling of being there for each other (Madianou and Miller 2012). This contemporary set of experiences is not equally available to all and is marked by the technological generational divide. Furthermore, ambient and continuous forms of copresence can be experienced as both an imposition and an invaluable source of care and support.[4] Transnational aged care in this context is potentially much more similar to aged care in proximate settings, in that family can be in touch as often as they desire, share the minutiae of everyday life and visit, if not regularly, at least when needed for crisis care.

In the two more recent cohorts, the circulation of distant care is facilitated by a high degree of choice of a range of ICTs available to the family members to use, albeit with varying degrees of different types of individual access. The potential provided by this polymedia environment can deliver a variety of effective forms of copresence experienced as a sense of "being there" for each other, despite the distance. New technologies, by increasing the sense of copresence across distance, also increase both the desire for and incidence of visits. At the same time, access to quicker and cheaper travel has increased the opportunity—and thus the pressure of obligation—to visit. Hence, the experience and practice of virtual copresence informs and impacts on that of physical copresence and vice versa. As I have argued elsewhere, it does not seem useful to argue about which is more important; the distinction appears arbitrary as the families in our study make use of all the forms of staying in touch across the distance that are available to them (Baldassar 2016b, 33).

NOTES

1. Whether these were in fact permanent repatriations or temporary visits is not known.
2. All but the first project benefited from funding grants from the Australian Research Council.
3. The White Australia Policy was the colloquial name for the 1901 Immigration Restriction Act, which refused entry to migrants who were not considered "white."
4. Relevant here is the burgeoning field that examines the plethora of *virtual* communities that can provide support as well as sites of activism and solidarity (see Karatzogianni and Kuntsman 2012; Kwan 2007).

PART THREE

Aging, Kin Work, and Migrant Trajectories

7

Returning Home

The Retirement Strategies of Aging Ghanaian Care Workers

CATI COE

Mabel Aboagyewa and Abena Frimpong[1] were migrants from Ghana who worked as home health aides in the United States for more than twenty years. When they retired from work in their early seventies, they returned to their hometowns in Ghana. This chapter explores the reasons why they did so, serving as an ethnographic example of the kinds of expulsions and exclusions in which states and capital are engaged and which individuals have to manage across their life courses.

In a recent book, Saskia Sassen (2014) argues that a new logic is emerging in the global political economy, the logic of expulsion. According to her argument, in advanced capitalism, "since the 1980s, there has been a strengthening of dynamics that expel people from the economy and from society, and these dynamics are now hardwired into the normal functioning of these spheres" (76). As profits are increasingly made from resource extraction and not from the production of goods and services, "people as consumers and workers play a diminished role in the profits of a range of economic sectors" (10). We need to examine what these expulsions and exclusions look like from the perspective of those who experience them, how they make sense of these exclusions, and the navigations they make in charting a pathway for themselves and others despite and through expulsion.

A retirement in Ghana for a worker in the United States is a kind of expulsion from the United States. Yet retirement in Ghana happens not through deportation or forced eviction, but through immigrant care workers' interpretations of their experiences with the aged in the United States and their anxieties about their own aged futures. Retirement in Ghana is not experienced as an expulsion, but as a logical choice—albeit one that is fraught and compromised.

Ghanaian elder-care workers in the United States find themselves in a paradoxical position as they themselves age: their work in nursing homes and home care reveal to them the impossibility of receiving the kind of care they have provided. Through their work, they are aware of nicer and private assisted-living facilities or home care, but know they cannot afford them due to their abysmal income as care workers. They are also aware of the overworked labor of nursing homes, and they do not want the lower quality care they could obtain through Medicaid in those sites. They would prefer family care, but their relatives in the United States, as labor migrants themselves, tend to be busy working and are therefore not available for unpaid care work (see Dossa, this volume). These options for an aged life in the United States produce anxiety. In response, many return to Ghana, where they feel that care by relatives is more available and elderly people are treated with respect.

The return to Ghana, however, is also marked by anxieties and affected by out-migration. Although they imagine home in certain ways, home is not quite the familiar place they expect. In Ghana currently, the kin most expected to give care are grown children, but the grown children of Ghanaian return migrants are usually also abroad, having followed or preceded their parents. Children, whether in Ghana or abroad, do tend to send remittances to support the care of their elderly parent, but the elderly rely on companionship and practical assistance from other kin nearby, whether siblings or the children of those siblings. Aging care workers work to nurture relationships with their kin in Ghana, meaning that they also give companionship as well as practical and financial assistance to these kin. Furthermore, although care workers' savings and Social Security go further in Ghana than they would in the United States, many rely on their entrepreneurship to earn additional money. They are therefore not solely recipients of care in their retirements, but also provide services and care in reciprocal ways as long as they can.

This chapter argues that the retirement strategies of Ghanaian care workers reveal how families and individuals are managing old age in an era of globalized capitalism, in which employers seek to shed their responsibilities for the care of workers and in which states are retreating from social welfare. I illustrate what expulsion on a global scale looks like ethnographically, and how a particular group of low-income workers in the United States manage their expulsion. In particular, I show how expulsion leaves people emotionally and financially vulnerable despite years of hard work. Nevertheless, people respond to expulsion creatively, even as the choices they make leave them somewhat disappointed and anxious.

Kin Work and Expulsion

According to Carol Stack and Linda Burton, kin work is "the labor and the tasks that families need to accomplish to survive over the life course" (1993, 157). Although kin work is often viewed as the unpaid care work done by family members, it is clear that families cobble together multiple resources to survive that include wage income; unpaid labor and gifts from kin, friends, and neighbors; and state-generated forms of support. Furthermore, Stack and Burton noted the important role played by nonkin and fictive kin in doing kin work. I want to extend the category of nonkin for care workers to include the state, nursing homes, home health agencies, and the clients of caregivers to suggest that they affect how the families of care workers sustain themselves over time in structuring the conditions of employment, including wage income. For example, in the United States, Medicare sets the rates at which care workers are paid, affecting rates in the private care market also. Historically, there have been exemptions in labor laws in this sector, for example in overtime pay and minimum wages, as the state has cared more about families' ability to hire care workers than care workers' ability to care for their own families (Boris and Klein 2012). Unions have been successful in fighting for higher wages in a few states and cities, but not in all, in part by convincing courts that the state—rather than private individuals or agencies—is the employer of record (Boris and Klein 2012; Mareschal 2006, 2007). Similar to the situation described by Delores Mullings (this volume), this employment environment affects homecare workers' ability to earn a wage that supports others, and to do kin work through sharing their income widely and generously with kin. How kin work is accomplished—how families sustain themselves over time—is affected by the conflictual and contested processes between capital, the state, and workers over the reimbursement and care of workers (Meillassoux 1972).

One historical example of how kin work is affected by the larger political economy is in colonial and apartheid South Africa. Here, the state constrained the movement of labor, restricting Africans' residence to selected areas, called homelands, the least fertile wastelands. Only those with an employment contract were allowed to live and work outside those areas. This regime resulted in men in the prime of their working lives migrating to factories and mines in the industrial belt and urban areas of South Africa, leaving behind their dependents—their elderly parents, their wives, and children—in the reserves, to scratch out a living from farming in the poor soils.

The result was translocal families. Those on the reserves were dependent on remittances from the migrants in the mines and cities. At the same time, those working were dependent on the reserves, for the industrial and commercial enterprises in the cities and mines did not provide adequately for these workers' retirement or disability. As a result, when workers were too old or sick to work any longer, they lost their employment contracts and had to return to their "homelands" (Mamdani 1996; Meillassoux 1981; Murray 1981; Schapera 1947). Anthropologist Claude Meillassoux concludes, "Preservation of the relations with the village and the familial community is an absolute requirement for the wage-earners, and so is the maintenance of the traditional mode of production [farming] as the only one capable of ensuring survival" (1972, 103). Businesses in South Africa were relieved of the responsibility of sustaining an individual laborer over the course of his or her life and for developing the next generation of workers. Instead, some of the costs were realized by those who remained in the reserves who took care of the elderly, sick, and disabled, and raised the children who would grow up to be labor migrants like their fathers. Furthermore, the human costs of such a system remained less visible because they were geographically distant.[2] Workers' maintenance of kin relations across distances accompanies the state's regulation of workers' mobility and residence as a way that families sustain themselves under conditions of exclusion.

One of the responses to expulsion within a political economy dominated by capitalism, therefore, is to rely on noncapitalist domains, such as relationships and obligations with kin, or what Neda Deneva (this volume) calls kinfare. Kin distribute economic resources through exchanges governed not by markets or by the desire for profit, but by emotional feeling, obligation, and reciprocity; that is, through alternative modes of valuation (Folbre 2008, 2001; Sahlins 2004; Zelizer 2005). These distributions are often not commodified, but occur through entrustment. In the words of Parker Shipton, "entrustment implies an obligation, but not necessarily an obligation to repay like with like, as a loan might imply. Whether an entrustment or transfer is returnable in kind or in radically different form—be it economic, political, symbolic, or some mixture of these—is a matter of cultural context and strategy" (2007, 11). Thus, among many Ghanaians, the care one received in childhood from one's mother, for example, creates entrustments to care for one's mother as an adult, including by sending remittances to her. Giving and receiving cash and care generate reciprocities and obligations in relationships, and it is the negotiation of these exchanges which cause the making, maintenance, and breaking of kin relationships (Coe 2011). Because gifts generate and maintain reciprocal relations, it is difficult to determine who is the beneficiary or recipient, and who the benefactor or giver, in kin work. The aged are not simply recipients of care or cash; rather, their kin work in the past may have created an entrustment that others reciprocate in the present. Because entrustment operates according to a different logic than capitalism or paid labor, it can serve as a safety net for individuals ill served by exchanges and relations dominated by capitalism.

Care workers in the United States face a similar problem to the mineworkers in colonial and apartheid South Africa: their low wages result in their inability to earn or save enough to ensure maintenance across their life courses in the place where they work. While Filipino care workers in Los Angeles wonder whether they will ever be able to retire (Nazareno et al. 2014), Ghanaian elder-care workers, facing a similar dilemma, respond by laying the groundwork to retire in Ghana. Ghana becomes a reserve to the United States, in the way that the homelands became to the industrial, metropolitan, and commercial agricultural areas of South Africa. How kin work is distributed across people in time and space, including transnationally, derives in part from the context of social welfare and employment options that are the result of national and transnational contestations between governments, capital, and labor. Ghanaians' migration from Ghana was similarly affected by these forces, even as they impel their return to the Ghana in their old age.

Ghanaian Migration: Past and Present

Transnational migration has been a known and valued phenomenon in Ghana since the colonial era: Ghanaians traveled for work elsewhere in West Africa and for education in Britain, processes that continued after independence (Goody 1982; Hill 1963). International migration from Ghana to Britain was once a sign of elite status, particularly when it accompanied a high-status education (Sekyi 1974). However, migration from Ghana increased in the 1980s and 1990s as structural adjustment programs in response to a prolonged economic crisis weakened the state's ability to provide needed services and enhanced the export-oriented segments of the economy. This focus on exports did not create many options for high-paid work, and cuts to government spending resulted in a decline in living standards for middle-class professionals and civil servants. International and regional migration increased as Ghanaians traveled to Nigeria and Libya at first (Twum-Baah, Nabila, and Aryee 1995), but now every country in the world that is economically better off is a potential destination—although the United Kingdom and the United States dominate migrant destinations outside Africa. It is estimated that between 3 and 7 percent of Ghana's population has migrated abroad (Twum-Baah 2005; World Bank 2011).

Although the middle class were the first to emigrate, as international migration increased in the 1980s and 1990s, the opportunity to travel became "democratized" (Manuh 2006, 24) in that a broader swath of the population, including students, teachers, lower-level civil servants, and skilled blue-collar workers like mechanics and electricians, has become increasingly involved in transnational migration. Some Ghanaian immigrants come to the United States with a green card obtained through the Diversity lottery; others overstay a visitor's or student visa. Those with a green card have better and more varied employment opportunities, but both authorized and unauthorized Ghanaian migrants end up working in elder care, the authorized in nursing homes and through home health agencies, and the unauthorized working "privately," contracted directly by a family to care for an elderly relative.

As international migration has expanded, it has become more characterized by struggle. The fruits of migration have shrunk for migrants, both because the cost of living has increased in Ghana, in part due to migrants' remittances, and also because of the kinds of jobs, such as in home care or retail, that these so-called unskilled migrants do abroad. Moreover, since Ghanaians are relatively recent migrants to the United States, they usually do not have an extensive family network to help with childcare and housing.[3] Thus, the return retirement migrations I describe below may just be a phenomenon of a first generation of transnational migrants, and not be the option that their children will choose. This same phenomenon may account for why Ghanaian care workers return home after postponing retirement, while Filipino care workers, in similar circumstances, talk much less about return migration. I turn now to discussing how elder care became a niche employment field for Ghanaians in the United States.

Ghanaians in Elder-Care Employment in the United States

Care work is a rapidly growing low-income occupation in the United States, and the experiences of aging care workers give us a sense of the pressures and anxieties other low-income workers in the United States face. Personal care and home health work are two of the top three fastest growing occupations in the United States (Bureau of Labor Statistics 2013), with the demand for services growing faster than the labor pool. This particular labor market is characterized by high levels of turnover (Wright 2005). Women comprise 89 percent of the elder-care workforce, and about half of the workforce are people of color (Smith and Baughman 2007). Surprisingly, given the physical demands of lifting another person, a substantial proportion of the workers are not young: 22 percent of the direct-care workforce is over the age of fifty-five (Paraprofessional Health Institute 2014).

In the early and mid-twentieth century, elder-care work was mainly done by African American and white immigrant women; and in the nineteenth century, by slaves and by domestic servants who were primarily immigrants from Europe (Glenn 1992). The legacy of servitude is visible in the current profession. As African American women found better employment opportunities in the wake of civil rights legislation in the late twentieth century, immigrant women (many of them recent immigrants) have replaced African Americans in this field, to the extent that in certain urban areas, they dominate it. In 2006, 20 percent of direct-care workers were foreign born (Khatusky et al. 2007; Smith and Baughman 2007). In metropolitan areas, in 2005, the proportion was higher: more than one in three nursing aides were foreign born (Redfoot and Houser 2005).

Immigrants in the United States tend to become concentrated in particular economic sectors within a segmented labor market, through their own social networks and employer ethnic stereotyping of workers (Lamphere, Stepick, and Grenier 1994; Waldinger and Lichter 2003). The fact that nursing aide work requires only a few weeks of training and is in high demand means that it is open and attractive to recent immigrants, whose education and work experiences may have been substantial in their own countries but require relicensing and retraining to pursue those same occupations in the United States (Choy 2003). With the increase in migration from Africa to the United States since the 1990s, new African immigrants have entered the field of elder-care employment disproportionately. In 2000, although only 2.8 percent of the total foreign-born population in the United States was from Africa, 11 percent of foreign-born nursing aides was African (Leutz 2007). My previous ethnographic research with the Ghanaian community in Philadelphia and more broadly along the East Coast found that health care is a niche employment sector for Ghanaians and other Africans—a self-reinforcing pattern, because their social networks help them find employment in the field.[4]

Nursing aide and home health work is considered unskilled, because one does not need a high school diploma, yet it requires a lot of emotional and social intelligence. Nursing aides are paid better than many other so-called unskilled occupations, but nonetheless many are working poor. Their median wages were $11.73 an hour, with an annual median income of $24,400 in 2012 (Bureau of Labor Statistics 2014). These low wages are primarily due to the role that Medicare and other forms of public funding play in determining compensation for direct-care workers (Boris and Klein 2012; Smith and Baughman 2007). Forty-six percent of direct-care workers rely on public benefits, and 16 percent have incomes that fall below the federal poverty line, a measure set so low that it underestimates the degree of poverty in the United States (Paraprofessional Healthcare Institute 2014). Like other poor people in the United States (Stack 1974), care workers are reliant on other forms of resource redistribution than through wage labor, such as the reciprocal relations of kin and state social-welfare schemes. Immigrant low-income workers have an option—namely, retirement to another country—which most nonimmigrant care workers would not consider.

The elder-care industry in the United States has become increasingly reliant on a migrant workforce because of the low wages, the emotional and social demands of the job, and the associations with historical servitude. Migrants find elder-care employment attractive because of the low-education threshold, the promise of regular employment, and their social networks, which help them find jobs in this field. However, the low wages make it difficult for workers to support their families. Like the Caribbean workers in Canada described by Delores Mullings (this volume), the poverty of care workers particularly becomes salient when it is time for them to stop working. For Ghanaian care workers, I argue, the nature of their work and the conditions of their employment encourages them to live transnationally by maintaining relationships with kin in Ghana and saving money for a business or a house, rather than planning to remain in the United States in their old age. In particular, they draw on their own experiences among the aged in the United States in thinking about their own aged futures.

The Figure of the Elder

Expulsion for care workers happens in part through the conditions of employment, particularly their low wages. However, when migrants talked to me about their decision to return home, they justified their decision through a different narration than expulsion. The interpretation of their social world that I heard over and over again from Ghanaian health-care workers was an idealization of the respect elderly obtain in Ghana. They base their decision on their perceptions of the ways that elder care is organized in the United States and Ghana. This recognition and justification set in motion certain actions that lead them to return to Ghana in their old age.

Ghanaian migrants, but particularly health-care professionals and elder-care workers with whom I discussed their lives and work, generally expressed the view that the elderly in America are not well cared for, in part because they live in institutionalized settings. The isolation of individuals and the segregation of age-grades across the life course in institutional settings is a product of how the state, families, and the market have shaped elder care in the United States. The employment of immigrants as elder-care workers is also a product of these interactions. The result is that immigrants tend to encounter elderly in the United States through their work, in institutions that can be isolating and bureaucratic, and that overload direct-care workers with too many residents to provide quality care.

In Ghana, in contrast, migrants emphasized that elderly were cared for by family members, even though anthropological and sociological studies have shown that families do not provide as much care as they are expected to (Aboderin 2004, 2006; Apt 1996; Dsane 2013; Van der Geest 2002, 1997). As Lawrence Cohen (1998) notes, the figure of the elderly person is good to think with, and among the migrants I encountered, it was used to contrast the United States to Ghana. Aging was nationalized by Ghanaian health-care workers: an elder hood at home could be enjoyed, but old age abroad was miserable.

Let me illustrate this point through a story told me by a live-in home health aide in her late forties. I had come to know Irene well through regular phone conversations over three years (2004–2007), when she mitigated the sense of constraint and claustrophobia while in her clients' homes by chatting with me. I also accompanied her on a visit to her house in Kumasi, where her children and parents stayed, for two weeks in August 2005. During my visit with her in Ghana, Irene told me about a conversation she had with a friend. Like many migrants, he had asked his mother in Ghana to handle the building of his house in Ghana, but, without his knowledge, his mother had put the house in his sister's name rather than his own. He found out what had happened on a visit home when his sister pushed aside his drying clothes on the clothesline, an action that led to an argument during which the truth emerged. He left Ghana after this incident, deciding that he would never return. Irene has similarly experienced conflict with her parents over her house, which they consider to be theirs. Despite pain over conflicts with her parents, Irene told her friend he would regret his decision to never live in Ghana again because she sees what the elderly in the United States experience through her work as a home health aide. "Only if you are middle class or upper middle class will you be okay in terms of nursing homes," she reported to me, and even then, "it is not nice." Her experiences of how the elderly are treated in the United States encouraged her to nurture ties with those in Ghana, despite feelings of anger and betrayal that otherwise might cause her, like her friend, to stay away.

These sentiments were echoed by others who similarly drew on their experiences in elder-care institutions in the United States to drive home their point about the difference between Ghana and the United States in terms of their treatment of the elderly. One nurse's aide in her sixties who worked in a nursing home told me that she would not want to end up in a nursing home: after seeing how the residents were treated, she would rather "jump off the roof." She said she had converted her nursing home colleagues so that the elderly were talked to respectfully, as they were in Ghana, as "Miss so-and-so" rather than simply by their first names. One man, who had worked as a nurse's aide in a nursing home while going to medical school, observed that the elderly in America are like "tissue paper," because they are "disposable." In Ghana, in contrast, he emphasized, the elderly are treated with respect. A third informant who worked as a nurse's aide in a neurological department of a nursing home talked about the lack of respect implicit in neglect, such as letting someone fall or not changing someone's diaper, when criticizing her colleagues. Thus, the United States was positioned as a sad place to be for an elderly person, because of the lack of

good care and respect one would receive, particularly in the institutional settings where these informants worked. Leslie Fesenmyer (2016) has described
a similar process of dichotomizing, essentializing, and nationalizing cultural
practices by Kenyan migrants in Britain, in which they consider Kenyans to care
for their families, unlike the British. Similar to Bengali elders in London (Gardner 2002), old age becomes associated with place, specifically, a pleasant old
age in the homeland and a sad old age in the country of migration. The dichoto-
mous thinking about old age influenced Ghanaian migrants to consider a return
migration in their retirement to be the best option.

   States play an important role in structuring these decisions. It is not that
the social support provisions for the elderly in Ghana are better than they are
in the United States, as one can argue is true for access to children's day care
(Coe 2012b). In fact, there is virtually no social welfare for the elderly in Ghana,
particularly for the vast majority who have worked in the informal sector as
traders or farmers (Doh 2012). It might then seem surprising that elderly Ghanaian immigrants would retire to Ghana. In the United States, social welfare for the
elderly is provided through Social Security and Medicare, the major programs by
which the American government fulfills its reciprocal obligations to its retired
workers and elderly population. As Neda Deneva (this volume) discusses also,
these programs function differently in enabling an elderly person's transnationalism. Social Security payments can be received by those who have worked in
the United States but live abroad—with some difficulty, but it is possible. Medicare payments, on the other hand, are limited to physicians and health-care
facilities in the United States. Greta Gilbertson's (2009) study of a multigenerational family from the Dominican Republic illustrates how elderly members
of this family receive Social Security payments in the Dominican Republic and
use them to support their own retirement and other members of the family.
However, those who wish to rely on Medicare had to visit the United States to
get medical treatment and pharmaceutical drugs. Because Social Security payments are pegged to one's income, those who earn a low wage, like home health
aides, earn very little in Social Security payments; contributory pensions like
Social Security do not benefit the poorest, who need a pension the most because
they lack other savings (Hennock 2007). It is difficult to live solely on Social
Security in the United States, but the cost of living is lower is Ghana.

   For Ghanaians, the low wages associated with elder care operate in two
contradictory ways: one, their income made return migration necessary; and
two, it pushed them into delaying retirement and return migration for as long as
they could. A person needed savings in order to ensure an honorable return to
Ghana. One could not return home empty-handed because relatives depend on
a migrant's savings, and starting a business or building a house is a sign of success. The low wages of elder-care work meant that aides could not save enough

to return home, and, like Filipino elder-care workers (Nazareno, Parreñas, and Fan 2014), delayed retirement until their bodies could no longer bear the physical strains of their work. On the other hand, the lower cost of living in Ghana meant that when one did (or had to) stop working and earning a wage, Ghana seemed like a better location in which to retire than the United States.

Ghanaian care workers' work experiences in the United States reinforce their sense that the United States is a place of sojourn, not a place to remain as an elderly person; a place to work, but not a place to receive care. As a result, America becomes associated with a particular stage in the life course—that of the working adult between the ages of twenty-five and fifty-five (Coe 2012a). It therefore plays a similar role that urban areas have played in Ghana historically, in which major cities have been places of temporary employment for young and middle-aged people whose hometowns function as a safety net, a place to return to in case of divorce or business failure (Brydon 1979; Caldwell 1969; Dei 1992). For immigrants in the United States, Ghana becomes idealized as a rural location where the elderly and children can receive good care, sometimes from each other.

The elder-care arrangements of the United States, which Ghanaians come to intimately know, seem impersonal, with vulnerable elderly at the mercy of disrespectful, overworked, and stressed workers and abandoned by their kin. Although the United States has far more generous provisions for the elderly than available in Ghana, the lower cost of living in Ghana and the transferability of Social Security payments across national borders make retirement in Ghana possible. Through migrants' imaginaries of old age and their actions on the basis of that analysis, Ghana has become a retirement community for Ghanaian-born care workers of America. In this chapter, I examine what expulsion through return migration felt like through the ambivalences and ambiguities of retirement for Mabel Aboagyewa and Abena Frimpong, two former home health aides.

Preparing for Retirement: Mabel Aboagyewa

I have known Mabel Aboagyewa for nine years, talking to her on the phone and accompanying her to social events in the Ghanaian diasporic community and among her network of friends and fictive kin in the United States. She has an outgoing, but not reflective, personality. I have gained a sense of her life through our conversations and visits, rather than through formal interviews in which she shared her life story. Through my visits, it seems to me that Mabel Aboagyewa, when she was not working in people's homes, had a life in the United States full of the warmth and vitality of longtime friends. I have also visited her in Ghana, two years after her return.

Mabel Aboagyewa came to the United States in 1964 as part of the World's Fair in New York City along with eight other young people from around the world. She was then in her early twenties. Although she told me that she had worked many jobs over her years in the United States, she worked, somewhat irregularly, as a live-in home health aide from the time I met her in December 2006 until her retirement in September 2013. She has no children and never married.

Because grown children are considered primarily responsible for providing financial support and care work to their elderly parents, being childless makes one particular vulnerable in old age. Many Ghanaians even consider it a tragedy. Mabel compensated for childlessness by staying very connected to her siblings and their children and by creating fictive-kin relationships and close friendships. Her nieces and nephews lived nearby in the United States; she made sure to stay in touch with them through phone calls and when she was home between live-in jobs. She also has a fictive daughter, the fifty-year-old daughter of a Sierra Leonean friend about her age; and several friends of Caribbean descent. She was appreciated in her local church whose congregation reflected the ethnic diversity of central New Jersey; its members gave her a very warm send-off that I was able to attend before she retired to Ghana.

In the United States, she lived in a decrepit basement apartment, shared with a relative of the owner, who lived upstairs on the main floor of the house. Like other live-in caregivers, she treated her residence as a place to stay between jobs, or a place to escape to when a job was not going well, not one in which to relax and make a life for herself. I visited her apartment several times. Her basement bedroom was filled with boxes of materials she was planning to take back to Ghana long before she returned. She kept these boxes in her bedroom because she was afraid that her roommate would steal her belongings if she left them outside her room. She did not keep toilet paper or any of her toiletries in the shared bathroom. She did not like to talk to me in the public spaces of the apartment because she was concerned about her roommate's mischief, and instead took me into her bedroom to sit on her bed and chat. Despite the wealth of social ties she had accumulated in her community, her residence in the United States seemed temporary because of the atmosphere of claustrophobia and paranoia. Her one safe space, the bedroom, was filled to the brim with appliances, clothes, and objects that served as a constant reminder, at least to me, that she was returning to Ghana and had gifting obligations to her relatives and friends there.

She started to speak with excitement about her return home as she approached the age of sixty-five, saying she would then be eligible to receive Social Security. However, she kept delaying the date of her departure, telling me each year for six years that she would go in September, before she actually left in September 2013 at age seventy. September was the month in which to return because her hometown's annual festival, which she wanted to attend, was celebrated during that time. When she left, she was in good health, but age was clearly making it harder for her to do the physical labor of caring for a frail or bedridden elderly person. She was walking more slowly, I noticed, and preferred to sit rather than stand. Her retirement from paid employment coincided with her return to Ghana.

When she retired to Ghana, she returned to a family house in her hometown in the Eastern Region, where she had grown up but had not been for forty-nine years, not even for a visit. She had not managed to build a home of her own, the dream of many migrants and a sign of success. Many Ghanaians would prefer not to live in a room in the family house, because living with other kin can create tensions. However, many middle-aged and elderly women do end up living in the family house after the loss of a job or end of a marriage. The family house functions as a safety net for family members, and they do not pay rent for their rooms. In her hometown in Ghana, Mabel was respected as a senior woman in the royal family, as her nephew is a powerful chief. But because of her long absence, she is not well known. She told me after a year there, in September 2014, that other people thought she had money because of her so-called pension (Social Security), but in fact, it was not a lot of money, she complained.

Her younger brother was very helpful to her immediately on arrival, taking her around, but he died suddenly about eight months after she arrived. Her older half sister, with whom I am also close, commented that it was a huge loss for them all, but particularly for Mabel, because she had been so practically and emotionally connected to him. The older sister remembered Mabel being quite downcast at the brother's funeral and seeing Mabel's face; the older sister wept, not for her own loss, but for Mabel's.

Mabel Aboagyewa was not entirely happy to be in her hometown, saying that there was a lot of gossip and she did not know whom to trust. She had made friends with an old schoolmate, another friend of mine, who commented to me that Mabel Aboagyewa was very American in her mannerisms and speech and was having trouble readjusting to life in her hometown. Perhaps as a result of her ambivalence about life in Ghana, right after her brother's funeral, Mabel returned to the United States for three months on an already planned visit, ostensibly to see her doctors and arrange her prescriptions because she was only allowed a three-month supply. Unfortunately for me, her visit to the United States coincided with my visit *to* Ghana in May-July 2014, but after my return, in September 2014, I was able to see her during a party to celebrate the birthday of the mother of Mabel's fictive daughter, with whom she stayed during her visit. At the party, Mabel brought out dresses sewn from wax print cloth and tie-dye in elaborate styles from Ghana to sell to her friends and neighbors. She did not have many buyers, but she was an aggressive seller and it was clear that the extra income was important to her.

Thus, Mabel prepared for many years to return to Ghana, making her home in the United States physically uncomfortable as a result. And yet she delayed retirement, perhaps anticipating the financial and emotional difficulties she would face despite her excitement about going home. Over her forty-nine years in the United States, she had developed a wealth of social ties, which, after two years' return, she had not yet duplicated in Ghana. Furthermore, she was under pressure from relatives and friends in Ghana to be financially generous because of her perceived wealth as a return migrant with her pension. Perhaps as a result of the ambivalences of her retirement in Ghana, after a year, she came for a long three-month visit to the United States to see her doctors and old friends, staying with her fictive daughter and celebrating the birthday of her daughter's mother. However, her financial constraints make such visits difficult. If such visits could pay for themselves through her selling Ghanaian clothes to her friends in the United States, then perhaps she could return more regularly and maintain a life on both sides of the Atlantic Ocean. Examining Mabel Aboagyewa's retirement, then, we see that expulsion is characterized by disappointment and ambivalence.

A Retirement in Ghana: Abena Frimpong

I met Abena Frimpong in July 2014 in another town in the Eastern Region, through the Presbyterian Church's aged fellowship group. After a long conversation with the fellowship group in which Abena Frimpong mentioned her situation, I returned with her to her house where we had an hour-long conversation in a mixture of Twi and English about her migration and retirement. At the time I met her, she was eighty-two years old; she was in good health, looking about ten years younger. She and her husband had divorced a long time ago, after thirteen years of marriage. She had trained as a midwife in Ghana, but never worked as one. All of her five daughters migrated abroad, and Abena Frimpong came to the United States in midlife, brought by one of her daughters who had just had a baby and wanted her mother's assistance with the newborn, like the grandmothers mentioned in the chapters by Deneva and Yanqiu Rachel Zhou (both in this volume).

Soon thereafter, Abena Frimpong wanted to begin earning money to care for her own mother, showing how kin work can be accomplished through remittances obtained through paid employment. She said, "My mother was alive, I had to do something [meaning, earn money]. . . . I had to work and look after my mother because my mother helped me so I had to help her. . . . She took care of my schooling so I promised my mother to take care of her."[5] She went to work as a home health aide, sometimes live-in and sometimes live-out, but preferring live-in work because the cost of transportation reduced her wages even further. She found home care to be very difficult work. During her years abroad, both her parents passed away, in the care of her siblings who remained in Ghana.

She returned to Ghana when she was seventy-two years old because she felt that America was not welcoming to old people, a common view of Ghanaians in the United States, as I have discussed above. "What is the use? America is not a place where they respect old people. *Eei* [a sound of horror/surprise]! So I thought, 'NO! I have to go home.' So I organized—I worked hard to earn money and I shipped my things home. I did everything all by myself [meaning, I took care of all the costs of my return; no one helped me]."[6] Once she decided that she was going home, she planned her return to Ghana over several years. She sent money to her sister to buy a plot of land in her hometown and she saved up money to build the modest house in which we were then speaking.[7]

Abena Frimpong has been living in her hometown for ten years. She survives on her Social Security payments—her pension from the American government, as she calls it. She admits that her major problem in retirement is loneliness. "Your children leave you."[8] She is old, so her children should be around her, she said. "It is painful." She complained that it was hard to catch up with her daughters through the internet (Skype) and by phone, as they are busy. "So it is difficult to get them."[9]

To compensate for her children and grandchildren's absence, she found other children to mother, like the grandmothers who foster children in China (Raffety, this volume). She opened a nursery for the emotional satisfaction of having people around. "When I came here, I said to myself, 'Oh, I am alone, and my children are not around.' Up until now, no one has come home. So I am alone. So I said, 'Let me do something to keep busy.' So I opened a small nursery [day-care center] in my house. I have expanded the school since, and that's what I do to keep busy [or, to amuse myself]."[10]

In the discussion with the aged fellowship group at her church, which I attended earlier in the day, another member of the aged fellowship commented on her nursery.

MAN: *εkanyan wo.* [It makes you feel lively.]

ABENA: *εkanyan me.* [It makes me feel lively.]

MAN: *εma wo hu nnipa.* [It allows you to see people.]

ABENA: *εma me hu nnipa; εma me hu mmɔfra. Kwee kwee, kwaa kwaa, Kwee kwee, kwaa kwaa, yee yee, yee yee yee yee, yee yee. εbεbɔ na obiara afiri me fie hɔ na aka me nkoa. εna mede gu so a mede te.* [It allows me to see people; it allows me to see children. (She makes noises representing the liveliness of the children:

Kwee kwee, kwaa kwaa, Kwee kwee, kwaa kwaa, yee yee, yee yee yee yee, yee yee).
At 3 P.M., everyone leaves and I am alone again. That's what I do to continue living.]

Indeed, when I visited her, the courtyard of the house was filled with the sounds of the toddlers who were just receiving a midday meal from four young female teachers. One of the toddlers wandered into the living room during our conversation, which made Abena Frimpong laugh, although she told him to return to the courtyard and the other children.

Although the nursery was satisfactory from an emotional point of view, from a financial perspective it has not been successful, because parents do not pay school fees on time. As a result, she was in debt, about which she complained bitterly. The nursery shows how difficult it is to see who is benefiting from whom: Abena provides a useful service in the community—a nursery—from which she derives energy and satisfaction on a daily basis and from which she hopes to earn a profit. Yet, like other business owners operating in Ghana, she extends credit to her customers and therefore is at real risk of not being able to sustain the business, particularly in her hometown where people may have claims to receive favors and gifts from her. In these circumstances, it is not clear who is helping whom: she is not simply the beneficiary of the children's energy but also creates the context for that energy to be expressed.

Another sign that she was not quite as alone as she felt was that during our hour-long conversation: her sister's daughter dropped by. The niece lives nearby in the family house with her mother; she also helps with the school. She said she came by a lot; she could do so "uninvited," she said. "I pop in." Abena Frimpong feels lonely, because her own children and grandchildren are far away and communication across that distance is difficult. However, she does have family nearby, and she has filled her house with the sounds of young children to stand in for her absent children and grandchildren.

From both life stories, then, we see the ways that aging care workers attempt to create a satisfactory retirement for themselves by returning to Ghana. Such a retirement means years of preparation and scrimping in the United States, including filling one's bedroom with boxes in the United States, in the case of Mabel Aboagyewa, and saving to build a house, in the case of Abena Frimpong. Because of their low wages, retirement was postponed until their early seventies. Social Security was essential to their retirement strategies, but they also worked to supplement it with additional sources of income.

Although retirement in the United States looks impossible (recall Abena's emphatic "NO! I have to go home!"), retirement in Ghana also has its share of disappointment and vulnerability, not always anticipated. Return migration takes them away from the social networks that they sustained during their migration:

for Abena Frimpong, her daughters and grandchildren; for Mabel Aboagyewa, her nieces and nephews, fictive kin, fellow congregants, and neighbors. Yet they found that there were family and friends in Ghana who were willing to be helpful. Abena Frimpong, who has been back much longer than Mabel Aboagyewa, has creatively started a business which makes her feel less lonely but not more financially secure, and Mabel Aboagyewa is trying to use her interest in fashion to create a small, cross-Atlantic business in Ghanaian-made clothes. They are recipients of care through the entrustments that they have generated over time, but, particularly in the case of Abena Frimpong, they also are business owners who provide services to others in their communities.

Conclusion: Understanding Experiences of Expulsion through Retirement Strategies

Kin work, or the labor of sustaining families over time, takes place through multiple channels, including the unpaid labor and entrustment of kin, wage employment, and state social welfare payments. The low rate of pay for elder-care workers does not promise a positive elderly future in the United States. Furthermore, it results in their having a harder time returning to Ghana as successful migrants with money to distribute to support their families and a house in their name. As a result of their low wages, they become more dependent on the trust fund of Social Security and entrustment of kin, to which and to whom they have contributed in the past. Their relatives in Ghana are particularly important for providing practical assistance and emotional companionship in retirement.

Aging Ghanaian care workers feel the dynamics of expulsion as they make choices about managing their life after paid employment. These choices are made using their interpretation of the lives of the aged in Ghana and the United States, in which their own work experiences with the elderly in the United States loom large. They use the figure of the elderly person to imagine their own retirement and nationalize old age: the elderly are given respect in Ghana, but are tossed away like used tissue paper in the United States. This view is surprising given the far more generous social welfare supports for the elderly in the United States than are available in Ghana, but their imaginary of old age in the United States is developed through their day-to-day work in elder care in which the elderly are taken care of by strangers, rather than kin, and usually in institutional settings driven by medical, bureaucratic, and financial constraints. Their retirement strategies have been structured by the negotiations between capital, governments, and workers' movements that have shaped old age care in the United States.

Through these imaginaries and interpretations of old age, then, Ghana becomes the retirement home or labor reserve for Ghanaian-born workers of the United States. It is here that they try to create a sense of self-worth and a home. Examining expulsion at a more microlevel, at the level of the individual, reveals how their dignity and creativity shines through despite their losses. Disappointed but managing, ambivalent about their situation but creative in response to their dilemmas, they cobble together different kinds of resources through kin and Social Security to make a home in Ghana in their old age.

ACKNOWLEDGMENTS

My thanks to the chairman and ministers of the local presbytery for organizing the fellowship aged group where I met Abena Frimpong. The research was funded by the Research Council and the Dean's Office of the Camden School of Arts and Sciences at Rutgers University. Rogers Krobea Asante was invaluable with his work on transcriptions, including that for the interview with Abena Frimpong.

NOTES

1. All names are pseudonyms.
2. As Cindy Hahamovitch describes with guest-worker programs in the United States, "By hiring a young, male labor force, agricultural employers banished the most persistent and media-worthy problems that had plagued the nation's fields since the late nineteenth century—child labor and illiteracy, abysmal maternal health care, and aged former farmworkers. They did so not by solving these problems but by outsourcing them to the United States' poorest neighbors" (2011, 8–9).
3. In response, they have developed fictive kinship networks, particularly through churches (van Dijk 2002) and hometown associations. Many Ghanaians abroad work long hours in difficult and low-paying jobs, making their ability to contribute to and benefit from these organizations precarious.
4. This finding is supported by wider survey data: 10 percent of those born in Ghana who were surveyed by the 2006–2008 American Community Survey worked in the healthcare industry in general, and another 8 percent worked in the single occupational category, as defined by the Bureau of Labor Statistics, of "nursing, psychiatric, and home health aides" (American Community Survey 2006–2008, my analysis).
5. The original: "My mother was alive, I had to do something [meaning, earn money]. . . . I had to work and look after my mother because my mother helped me *enti ɛsɛsɛ me nso meboa no. . . . ɔhwɛɛ me sukuu enti na ma* promise *me maame sɛ mɛhwɛ no.*"
6. The original: "What is the use? America *nso nyɛ kuro a yɛbɔ aberewa anaa akɔkoraa wɔ mu oow. Eei! Enti ɛbaa m'adwene mu sɛ,* 'NO! I have to go home.' *ɛna mesiesie—mebɔɔ mmɔden yɛɛ me biribi a me*ship *me nnɔɔma.* I did everything all by myself."
7. Land in Mabel's hometown was more expensive than in Abena's hometown.
8. The original: "*Wo mma kɔgya wo.*"
9. The original: "*Enti eyɛ* difficult to get them."
10. The original: "*Mebaae no ɛna mese,* 'Oow, me nkoa ara, me mma no deɛ yɛamma bi.' Up till now *obiara amba. Enti me deɛ eyɛ me nkoa. Enti mese,* 'Oow, daabi, ɛsɛsɛ meyɛ biribi na mede gyegye me ani.' Enti me* gather *mmɔfra ɛna meyɛɛ* nursery *kakra w ɔ me fie. Enti seesei ɛno na megu so a mede regyegye me ani.*"

8

Balancing the Weight of Nations and Families Transnationally

The Case of Older Caribbean Canadian Women

DELORES V. MULLINGS

The historical significance of older Caribbean Canadian women's kin work remains relatively obscure in Canada. Canada has been blessed with a generation of Anglophone Caribbean women who have traveled and coexisted transnationally between their birth countries in the Caribbean and Canada, a place they also call home. Their strength and resilience cemented their success as Canadian citizens. This group of women have aged in place in Canada; the stereotypes about older adults, older women in particular, would suggest that these women require care and have become dependent on family and friends for their survival. However, Caribbean Canadian older women's lives contradict this myth. These women's gendered kin work in Canada began with their entrance into the West Indian Domestic Scheme in the 1950s and this kin work continued as they supported their families financially across borders through remittances. As the women age, the type of support and care they provide change. Where they once provided full financial support to children and kinfolk, now they are assisting by caring for young children and others religiously and culturally. Drawing on Critical Race Feminism as a theoretical orientation and critical race counter-storytelling as a methodology, I discuss and analyze the kin work of Caribbean Canadian older women.

I am implicated in this research as a product of the West Indian Domestic Scheme. My aunt Hanna (Amy), now deceased, whom I called Mom, came to Canada as a domestic worker in 1968. As an adolescent and young adult, I was privy to many of the stories that my mom and her Caribbean female friends shared among themselves. I am therefore invested in ensuring that their counter-stories are widely disseminated so that Canadians can have a better understanding of their history in Canada and their contributions in the

Caribbean and Canada. In addition, increased knowledge about this population can offer policy makers and service providers important information that will influence the care needs of these women.

The Context of Caribbean Immigration

The Caribbean is an eclectic mixture of many different groups of people. The majority are descendants of African slaves with substantial minorities of the descendants of Chinese and Indian indentured servants and European slave masters, business owners, and administrators (Beckles 1989). The devastation of the Caribbean region caused by mining (e.g., bauxite) and deforestation for sugar cultivation destroyed its natural resources and ultimately the relationship between the land and its people.

The colonial theft of natural resources, domination, and pillaging created the push factors of high unemployment and underemployment, a low standard of living, classism, shade-ism, and inaccessible postsecondary education that motivated Caribbean people to seek better and more prosperous lives in other parts of the world (Allahar 2010b; Beckles 1988, 1989; Chodos 1977; Foner 2009). Several authors in this volume (Coe, Yarris, and Zhou) cite poor economic conditions, neoliberalism policies, capitalism, and remnants of colonialism and imperialism as common reasons for women's and grandparents' motivation for migration, whether as caregivers for their own grandchildren or others in private homes or institutions. In the case of Caribbean Canadian women, the pull factors in postwar Canada were aligned with the needs of the Caribbean people. Canada's thirsty labor market needed skilled and unskilled laborers to support its growing economy. The Caribbean responded by supplying cheap labor—men as agricultural workers (Cecil and Ebanks 1992) and women as domestic workers (Calliste 1989, 1993a, 1993b; Daenzer 1993, 1997; Silvera 1989).

These immigration patterns continue unabated: immigrants have been a consistent and reliable source of cheap labor, which have fueled Canada's economy. Caribbean people have always been keen to work in Canada, often under some of the most exploitative, discriminatory, and unsafe conditions. Through one early program, one hundred Black women from Guadeloupe went to Montreal as domestic workers in 1911 (Calliste 1989). Strong activism from both Jamaican government officials and Canadian community-based advocacy organizations motivated Canada to initiate a formal domestic program in 1955, which allowed Black Caribbean women to enter Canada as domestic workers (Armstrong and Taylor 2000). Canada's West Indian Domestic Scheme was implemented until 1967, through which approximately three hundred Caribbean women were accepted into the program each year (Calliste 1993a; Daenzer 1992). The racist immigration policy ordered that applicants be tested for syphilis and stipulated that they had to be between the ages of eighteen and thirty, unmarried, and without children (Calliste 1993a, 1993b; Daenzer 1993, 1997; Silvera 1989) to be eligible for the program. As a result, many of the women did not document having children and partners in the Caribbean in order to qualify for entrance into Canada. The women's mothering roles and responsibilities were thus publicly denied.

Contrary to popular beliefs that Caribbean people were uneducated when they entered Canada, immigrants who arrived between the 1950s and 1970s had postsecondary education (Plaza 2004; Richmond 1993; Simmons and Plaza 2006). Brand (1991) tells the story of Marjorie Lewsey, a Canadian-born Black woman, who recalls: "My mom came to Canada, I believe, in 1919 from Baseterre, St. Kitts. She was a grammar school teacher in St. Kitts. You realize that Black women then, and, I guess, as now, had to come as domestics" (240). The majority of the women arrived as nurses and domestic workers under extremely hostile conditions.

Black women's sense of identity is strongly related to and aligned with mothering; therefore, in the absence of opportunities to mother directly, they created alternative mothering roles transnationally. Consequently, the women developed strategies to care for their children while living apart and in many cases other relatives such as grandparents, sisters, and aunts cared for their children while the women in turn assumed financial responsibilities for their children's caregivers. Erica Lawson explains that "motherhood and mothering practices are powerful aspects of how women" negotiate the challenges and complexities of an ever increasing globalized world. "From this perspective, transnational mothering and maternal politics were not just sites of resistance for" Caribbean women; they "also allowed them to enact embodied identities and construct communities away from home" (2013, 147). Historically, Caribbean women, like other Black women in the diaspora, have viewed child-rearing and motherhood as collective enterprises where "other mothers" from extended families and kinship networks assume some of the responsibility of mothering, known as child-shifting in the Caribbean literature (Collins 1994, 1997; Massey-Dozier 2011). Caribbean Canadian women had to draw on their extended families, often the children's grandmothers, to support their child-shifting arrangements when their families were disrupted. Neda Deneva (this volume) cites Arlie Russell Hochschild (2003) in describing this practice as care drain in which young immigrant women leave their families behind to provide care to children and older adults in wealthy countries. In the case of the Caribbean Canadian women, the physical disruption was replaced with transnational financial caring for offspring and families, one of the most important reasons the women immigrated to Canada. Kristin Yarris (this volume) also discusses intergenerational migration where daughters in Nicaragua, like the Caribbean Canadian women in this study, immigrate because of poor economic conditions in their countries and their mothers assume responsibilities for their children. For both groups of women, the negotiated caring along gendered lines is implicit both in the home country and abroad. In this way, sending remittances to care for family, especially children and extended family, was and still is commonplace and expected. While Nicaraguan migrant mothers send remittances to support mostly their children and their own mothers, for the Caribbean Canadian women, the remittances also served as a means to help prepare for their eventual return to their birth countries.

Critical Race Theory

I explore older Black Caribbean Canadian women's experiences of caring transnationally through a Critical Race Feminism (CRF) analysis using the methodology of counter-storytelling (Delgado 1988; Love 2004; Solórzano and Yosso 2001, 2002). However, since CRF is a splinter group of Critical Race Theory (CRT), I begin by discussing the premise of the CRT movement. Critical race theorists aim to transform racist social structures. To accomplish this goal, they have several tenets, which include locating racism at the center of their analysis and arguing that marginalized people must narrate their own experiences and realities (Ladson-Billings and Tate 1995). In addition, activists argue that racism is endemic and insidious and therefore produces and reproduces relationships of power, domination, and subordination (Villalpando and Delgado Bernal 2002). Furthermore, they "question the very foundation of the liberal order, including equality theory, legal reasoning, Enlightenment rationalism, and neutral principles of constitutional law" (Delgado and Stefancic 2012, 3). Proponents use case law, policies, and institutional conduct to demonstrate that institutional practice, government and organizational policies, the law and the legal process are color blind (Aylward 1999; Crenshaw 1989, 1995; Delgado 1995; Fernandez 2002; Gotanda 1991; Matsuda 1991; Solórzano and Yosso 2002; Williams 1991), what I refer to as color invisibility (Mullings 2015). Activists challenge the notion of meritocracy, suggesting that such an ideology represents a false sense of advancement. Furthermore, they argue that policy makers fail to institute reforms to change the course of institutional racism and, when changes are made, they are based on the principle of interest conversion or self-interest so that working-class whites benefit from such changes (Delgado 1995; Gotanda 1991; Matsuda 1991). The CRT movement has expanded beyond legal studies and now includes social issues such as education, employment, mothering, and immigration.

Racialized women felt that their concerns were minimized or excluded. They argued that the CRT movement focused more on men's issues (e.g., over-policing), and when women scholars addressed women's issues, their activism highlighted issues of importance to white middle- and upper-class women (e.g., abortion rights) and "if mentioned at all, the differing experiences of women of colour were often relegated to footnotes" (Wing 1997, 3). Similar to other gender-related discourse, white female legal scholars identified patriarchy as the main cause of women's marginalization in society (MacKinnon 1983, 1993) and predictably failed to acknowledge race in their activism and analysis (Turpel 1993).

Critical Race Feminism activists centralize racialized women's experiences and analyze those experiences based on their race and other identities, what Kimberlé Crenshaw (1989) calls intersectionality. We cannot reduce the lived experiences of older Black Caribbean women to one essential form; their experiences are situated along racialized, gendered, classed, immigrant status, and aged axes. Critical Race Feminism continues to grow as Aboriginal and racialized scholar-activists write about race-based marginalization on various topics from their unique perspectives (see Berry 2009; Evans-Winters and Esposito 2010; Few 2007; Houh and Kalsem 2015; Houle 2011; Verjee 2012). Critical Race Feminism, therefore, is an appropriate theoretical framework to explore the transnational caring roles of Black Caribbean Canadian older women because it focuses attention on their experiences of race, class, and gender using an intersectional lens to create a space for their voices to be heard through counter-storytelling.

Counter-Storytelling

Racism in Canada determines whose stories are seen as truth and who is identified as a legitimate Canadian. Historically stories about African Canadians are shaped by white perspectives; therefore, these "truths" determine the way in which Caribbean Canadian Black women are denied or have access to resources, how their bodies are represented in social institutions (e.g., media), and how others perceive them. Black people in Canada, and by extension older Black Caribbean Canadian women, are relegated to the margins of Canadian society, a position from which they have little group power; consequently, they rarely have institutional privilege and decision-making power. Therefore, stories about them are perpetuated by what Richard Delgado (1988) calls the "in group," who creates majoritarian stories based on their own experiences of power and privilege. According to Daniel G. Solórzano and Tara J. Yosso, "story-telling is racialized, gendered, and classed and these stories affect racialized, gendered, and classed communities" (2002, 32).

As an individual who has lived experience with racial and gendered subjugation, my first-person account is a requirement in counter-storytelling (Delgado 1988); therefore, as a Black woman of African Caribbean descent, my voice is important in helping to set the agenda for the Caribbean Canadian women's counter-stories. Counter-storytelling offers me the researcher a space to help the women share their stories. Parin Dossa and Cati Coe, in the introduction of this volume, introduce Noor's counter-story as an older Iranian woman who does embroidery work. Similarly, I have a responsibility to represent older Caribbean Canadian women's stories ethically and responsibly in their words as well as possible (Mullings 2004). I therefore use the women's words to represent their stories. For example, the term "partner" is more gender-neutral than "husband" to describe an intimate loved one; however, the women used "husband" to describe their loved ones during our conversations either generally or in reference to themselves. I use the term "husband" to honor the women's words.

In an act of resistance, I am using counter-stories to challenge the legitimacy and truth of the majoritarian stories about older Black Caribbean Canadians. Simultaneously, I am questioning the perspectives of the so-called in group as knowers and creators of knowledge about these older women. Furthermore, the counter-stories I will recount are those that older Black Caribbean Canadian women shared with me from their perspectives; creating this opportunity for the women to share their stories ensures that they shape the discourse around their lived experiences. I use counter-stories to destroy the perception of Black people in Canadian popular culture, which suggests that Blacks are newcomers to Canada (Bobb-Smith 2003), exploit and deplete the Canadian welfare systems, and have no affinity or commitment to the Canadian state (Allahar 2010a). Other African Canadians are using counter-stories to share their perspectives and create powerful tools to challenge the status quo and the centrality of white dominance. They share counter-stories about discrimination and exploitation in Canada in areas and institutions such as the criminal justice system (Aylward 1999); race, gender, and sexual identity (Silvera 1992); history (Cooper 2006); mothering (Mullings 2010, 2013); employment discrimination (Mullings 2015); identity and racial subjugation (Bobb-Smith 2003); Caribbean domestic workers (Daenzer 1992, 1997; Silvera 1989); and Black Canadian identity (Brand 1991). "Stories create their own bonds, represent cohesion, shared understandings and meanings" (Delgado and Stefancic 2000, 60). After discussing my methodology, I use CRF and counter-storytelling to explore older Black Caribbean Canadian caregiving and support roles.

Methodology

The research was guided by the following questions: What were the experiences of Black Caribbean women in the Canadian labor market? What are the financial realities of living in Canada after retirement? How do Black Caribbean women contribute to their families and communities? Using Rowland Atkinson and John Flint's (2001) process for accessing hard-to-reach populations, participants were recruited through purposive snowball sampling and they were prescreened for eligibility and suitability for the research project through initial telephone interviews. In-depth individual interviews were conducted in person with three people: two older women and one male community advocate. I also conducted a focus group with four women who requested a group interview and one combination e-mail and telephone interview with one female community advocate. Seven participants signed consent forms prior to their interviews and one gave an audio-recorded verbal consent. The individual interviews lasted approximately ninety minutes and the focus group lasted two and a half hours. All individual and focus groups interviews were audio-taped with permission from the participants and later transcribed verbatim. These were later member-checked with participants to ensure accuracy of the information. Transcripts were then analyzed thematically following Jennifer Attride-Stirling's (2001) five-step process.

I experienced a number of challenges associated with participant recruitment; hence, I had a smaller-than-expected sample for this pilot study. I canceled three confirmed interviews when two participants became ill and one left the country due to unforeseen circumstances; this reduced the diversity of the group of older women but gave me insight into how life transitions among older Caribbean women can happen suddenly and unexpectedly. I did not anticipate the focus group interview, however, four participants indicated that they wanted to be interviewed as a group; they noted feeling comfortable sharing their stories in the presence of others who had similar experiences. I explained to participants that confidentiality cannot be guaranteed in a group discussion but they felt fine to continue. I attempted to have participants from at least four countries in the Caribbean; however, in the end, Jamaica was overwhelmingly represented with five retired women and two advocates. A single participant came from another island, which will remain unnamed for confidentiality reasons. Statistically, Jamaica has a larger population in Canada than any other Caribbean island; therefore, it is not surprising that Jamaicans are heavily represented in this sample.

Findings

The sample consisted of eight Black, Caribbean-born participants (seven women and one man), six retired older women and two community advocates, who immigrated to Canada prior to 1969 and have worked in Canada for more than thirty years. However, for the purpose of this analysis, I will use only the data from the six older women. The data from the community advocates focused exclusively on labor laws, labor-related discrimination, and Canadian human-rights policies, which are beyond the scope of this paper. The six retired women were between the ages of sixty-nine and eighty-two with an average age of seventy-five. They worked in various places including hospitals, long-term care facilities, nursing homes, factories, people's homes, and department stores (see table 8.1). All six women entered Canada with postsecondary education or technical training; however, they did not all find work immediately (or ever) in their professions so they worked where they could find employment.

All the women live with various forms of chronic diseases, including high blood pressure, heart disease, hypertension, diabetes, renal failure, and glaucoma (see table 8.2). The women have a health profile associated with long-term poverty (Black 2000; Williams and Williams-Morris 2002).

At the time of the interviews, the women's incomes were a combination of Old Age Security (OAS), Canada Pension (CP), and Guaranteed Income Supplement (GIS).[1] Two participants, in addition, had personal savings to draw from. None of the women had Registered Retirement Savings Plans and two of the six women had a small amount of emergency savings. None had investments or income from employment.

All six participants in this study had been married; two were currently married. One woman became a single mother after her marital relationship dissolved and a second divorced after her children were grown; neither remarried or had any significant long-term relationships. One woman is a widow. Three of the women live with adult children and two women live with their husbands (see table 8.3). Five owned (single or jointly) the homes that they live in. These living arrangements are common in the Caribbean where most families cohabitate and support each other from birth to death.

Several themes emerged from the data; however, for the purpose of this chapter, I will focus on the women's financial needs in retirement and their

TABLE 8.1
Participants' Field of Employment

Industry	Number of women
Hospitals	4
Nursing homes and long-term care facilities	4
Private homes	3
Factories	2
Department store	2

TABLE 8.2

Participants' Health Concerns

Health concerns	Number of women
Diabetes	5
High blood pressure	3
Gastrointestinal disorder	3
Heart disease	3
Back pain	3
Kidney disease	2
Depression	2
Hypertension	1
Cataracts	1
Glaucoma	1
Hearing impairment/deafness	1
Stroke	0

TABLE 8.3

Living Arrangements and Marital Status

Living arrangements	Number of women
Live with husband	2
Live with children	3
Live alone	1
Marital status	
Married	2
Widowed	1
Divorced or separated	3

contributions to their families and communities through volunteering and religious participation. Each of the themes creates counter-stories to help make visible the women's transnational caring roles.

The Counter-Stories

As retirees, the women require the financial support of family members to remain in their homes. However, they provide significant support to their children, grandchildren, church community, and larger community by volunteering their time. They have created transnational communities in Canada but they continue to keep their Caribbean cultural values alive in various ways. After retirement, the women shifted caregiving roles to helping to parent their grandchildren and supporting their communities by participating in religious-based civic activities. The women also contribute to the larger society by volunteering in various not-for-profit and government institutions.

Counter-Story 1: Support to Family in Canada and the Caribbean

Pseudonyms are used to represent the six women who noted that when they were employed, they sent remittances to help with house repairs, the purchase of large items such as cars, airplane tickets for relatives to emigrate from the Caribbean, and small business equipment (e.g., sewing machines, storage containers, and farming tools). They helped to pay school fees for relatives' children and sent goods. Irene and Patsy recall sending barrels back home filled with gifts of clothing and shoes to their relatives.

> Me and the other girls [other Black Caribbean friends] used to go down to "rozzoe" [used clothing stores] and pick up things for the barrel. Nice new things you never know that people give wey [away] those things but dem [those] days it was cheap. [She sucks her teeth in what is known as "kiss teeth" in the Caribbean.[2]] You should see the kind of things we used to get fi [to] put ina de [into the] barrels. Nice man. (Magg)

> I send barrels to Mama two time ah year with clothes for everyone, food, shoes, and everything that them needed. Every year. Mi used to start collecting tings fi de [next] barrel right after mi post the last one. (Kat)

In addition to sending goods, some sponsored children and other kinfolk and cared for them financially and materially until they left their homes or became financially independent, as other studies have described (Crawford 2003; Lawson 2013). Mar sends "money to my sister to help with her grandchildren. The daughter noh [don't] have it and one ah the likkle bwoy [one of the little boys] really bright [smart] so we try to help."

Similar to Frances Henry's (1994) findings, the women discussed building homes and investing in property and small businesses back home so maintaining relationships was and continues to be an important activity even if the dream of returning home is unrealized. My mom Hanna returned to Jamaica eight months of each year as a part of her retirement plan. Some of the women in this study also planned to return home to their birth countries after retirement; however, their plans have not materialized. Aging in place has also necessitated that the women find different ways to care for and support their children. The women provide support to their immediate families in Canada primarily as caregivers in various capacities. Eny said: "I carry my granddaughter to her lessons three times a week. She is busy taking all kinds of lessons. Piano, violin, and acting. Some days it's tiring too because you know I am tired and when it is really cold, I don't really want to go out but if I didn't go I don't think [name] would get to go to her lessons you understand."

Yanqiu Rachel Zhou (this volume) discusses the incorporation of older Chinese immigrants into the global economy as unpaid childcare providers. Similarly, as grandparents, the women in this study are now helping to mother and parent their grandchildren without state enumeration or recognition. In Zhou's study, the grandparents emigrated from China in later years while the older adults in this study have aged in place. Nonetheless, both groups of older adults are providing free care in Canada for their families. Although the older Caribbean Canadian women are not parenting full-time, like some of the Chinese grandparents in Zhou's study, child-shifting has occurred so they assume responsibilities for taking children to participate in extracurricular activities and caring for them in the home. Historically, Caribbean grandmothers have assisted in caring for their grandchildren even when there is no family disruption. These older women had child-rearing support from their own mothers and other kinfolk when they immigrated to Canada in search of better lives.

Some women's transnational caring and caregiving shifted from the Caribbean to Canada, but it is also evident that some women continue to care for their kinfolk who remain in the Caribbean through remittances. Sending remittances is an expectation held by others left behind and considered by immigrants as a responsibility, but maintaining contact with family and friends is also important to the women themselves, especially when they envision returning home after they amass their fortunes and retired. Cati Coe (this volume) discusses Ghanaian care workers returning to Ghana as a retirement plan, but she also addresses the breakdown of relationships with their children who are often still living in the United States. All the women in this study remained in Canada and have close contacts with their children, but it is interesting to note that they remain in Canada because they could not afford to return to the Caribbean, not having saved enough to sustain themselves. Staying in touch with others back home was deliberate to create a sense of identity, feelings of belonging, and cultural continuity as evident in the many displays of transnationality in food and culture (Chamberlain 1998). The women have successfully kept their cultures alive in Canada and created subcultures representing a rich combination of Caribbean and Canadian cultures.

Their transnational culture also includes mothering, which is essential to their sense of identity. As noted previously, child-rearing and mothering are seen as collective responsibilities to be shared among kinfolks, and they continue with this tradition (Collins 1994, 1997; Massey-Dozier 2011). The caring, however, has shifted so that the women developed two sets of kinship networks: one in Canada and one in the Caribbean, in which they simultaneously perform caring and mothering roles and responsibilities. The women also contribute to their communities by volunteering in various capacities and through their religious involvement.

Counter-Story 2: Financial Well-being

Statistics Canada (Townson 2005) found that older women tend to be poorer than older men, but when women cohabit with others their poverty rates decrease. This theme is evident among the older women in my study: the women need less financial support when they reside with partners or children. High financial obligations to those at home, as discussed in the previous section, meant that these women were less likely to prepare adequately for retirement. In addition, given that they earned less than their white women colleagues (James 2009), these women were put at a disadvantage with respect to the amount of retirement income they are entitled to. If they live with others, they are likely better off financially. Coe (this volume) also argues that the wages earned by retired Ghanaian care workers in the United States were insufficient to sustain them across their life course in the United States, so the retirees use Ghana as a reserve. Similarities between the Ghanaian retired care workers and Black Caribbean Canadian older women further emphasize how Black care workers are used to sustain a global economy and then discarded when they can no longer care for mostly white children and older adults.

The women discussed their need for financial support from family to have an adequate standard of living and remain in their communities in Canada. One woman clearly stated that she could not manage without her daughter's help; she said, "Right now I live wid [with] my daughter and I don't know how I would manage if I didn't have help." The same theme reverberates for another who noted that she "don't have any problem because living with the children help a lot. Everybody contribute to paying the bills and I can buy what little things I need for myself." Ver lives alone and therefore, of the six women, experiences the greatest financial stress. She said, "It's tough, it's very tough. Sometimes I can't buy no food to eat after I pay the $980 for rent. After I pay the bills there is nothing left. I go down to my daughter to get food." Ver needs additional income even with her Canada Pension funds and other government supplements. She was unable to save for retirement and had not been employed at any time with an employer who paid benefits so she has no other source of income. Magg is more financially secure than Ver; she owns the house in which she lives and she receives rent from her child with whom she lives. Even so, she feels financially stretched and relies on family support and informal employment. She said: "The mortgage is high on the house and the taxes are high too. I can't pay all the bills so I take in—you know—a little babysitting to help with the bills. I was trying to find a part-time job to help out but—you know—dem [they] think dat [that] me too old so nobody noh waan fi hire mi [no one wants to hire me]. If I didn't have help from mi children I don't know how I would manage."

Four of the six participants experience financial stress and would have difficulty remaining in their homes if they lived alone or did not have the support of their children. Ver, the only individual who lives alone, faces hardship and, as she noted, after paying her rent, she cannot afford to purchase food. One woman who was doing okay said, "We are okay because my husband get his pensions and I get my own too. The two of us together make it easier and the mortgage on the house is low so we don't have a lot of expenses. Ongle [only] when something have to fix tings get a likkle tight—you know what ah mean?" (Eny).

Women were more financially secure when they worked full-time. One woman traveled extensively to her birth country while she was employed; however, that lifestyle has changed since her retirement. Although she can afford most necessities, she can no longer afford to travel. Another woman discusses her financial limitation: "I can buy my food and my meds but I can't afford fi [to] travel to Jamaica like when I was working yuh understan [do you understand]? I doan [don't] have a penny to mi name aside from wha de government give me every month."

One may argue that older white women in Canada are in similar positions. But older Black Caribbean Canadian women did not enjoy equal pay for work of equal value and might be better off in retirement if they were properly financially compensated, especially given that they were always employed. Participants have worked all their lives but rely on financial support from family, and some continue to work informally, an indication of the weakness of social support in Canada. Although the women in this study depend on cohabitating with their children to survive financially, they are not as dependent on their children like the grandparents in Zhou's research study. They have lived in Canada for most of their lives so they are eligible for Old Age security on their own merits given that they exceed the minimum ten years' residency requirement. The Caribbean Canadian women's financial circumstances offer them more freedom than their Chinese counterparts. This freedom provides them with the ability to engage in religious institutions in various ways.

Counter-Story 3: Religious Engagement

Religion as a form of spirituality is important to all the women in the study. The significance of religion and the church for Caribbean Canadians seems similar to the role of the Black church in Canada (see Este 2004). Data about African Caribbeans' religious engagement in Canada is limited so a much more extensive literature about Black Caribbean people in the United States will be used to help support my analytical arguments. Linda Chatters and her colleagues (2008, 2011) assert that Black Caribbeans utilize religion as a coping mechanism and social support. Robert Joseph Taylor and his colleagues found that "Caribbean Blacks indicated high levels of organizational religious participation, strong endorsements of the subjective religiosity items, as well as reports of private prayer" (2010, 12).

Barring illness, all the women attend church services at least twice a week, usually on Sundays and once during the week for prayer meetings. They attend other gatherings such as fasting, special services (e.g., women's or seniors' ministry activities), funerals, and conventions. In addition, the women have specific roles in their churches as prayer mothers or women who lead special prayer services for people in need, choir members, and evangelists or church members who minister to people in the community outside of church hours.

I argue that these religious activities represent women's ongoing attempts at adaptation and transformation of religious traditions. These are normative activities and roles in Caribbean churches; the women have adapted to Canadian society by transferring these cultural values and activities to their lives in Canada. For example, two informants talked of their prayer groups attending nursing homes and prisons. The women note that even those in nursing homes still minister to others by offering prayers to sick individuals. "My church have a prison ministry and we go in to talk with the prisoners and tell them to be of good cheer. You know it's hard for them to be in those places right, so when we go we carry likkle [little] care packages of food and tings [things] like dat [that] right" (Ethel).

This finding is similar to Alex Stepick, Terry Rey, and Sarah J. Mahler (2009) and Robert Joseph Taylor, Linda M. Chatters, and Jeff Levin (2004) who found Caribbean Blacks in the United States are similarly engaged in their religious communities. The women commit to their church financially. Mar said: "Yes, I throw my tithe every month, even if I don't have it I make sure I pay it because that is how you get blessings. The Bible tell us that we have to pay our tithe 10 percent of your income so no matter what likkel [little] me have, me mek [make] sure dat me pay mi tithe."

When there is a death in the church, church members take up a collection of money that is known as a "love offering" to be given to the grieving family. In situations where they are unable to donate money to members of the church, they find creative ways such as providing food to church members and their extended families. "When we have a death ina de [in the] church we pick up love offering to help the family so I always give a likkle something. Even if I don't have anything that month I cook and bake and bring to the family to help feed the people that gather at the dead house" (Ver).

The women demonstrate the traditional Caribbean cultural fabric of blending religion and spirituality in daily life in the roles that they occupy in the church and the responsibilities that they assume even when they are unable to support church activities financially.

Counter-Story 4: Community Contributions

The women support the small Caribbean Canadian communities through their religious, social, and familial activities, but they also contribute to the larger Canadian society by volunteering in various organizations, including food banks, a center for older adults, and hospitals, and in these ways show their transnational orientation. "The food bank that I used to go to need a lot of help so I volunteer there twice a week. One of my friend used to volunteer there and that is how I get to know of the place. You know even though I can't give food a lot of time I like to go to give a little something. My time is something right" (Ver).

One participant said she volunteered at the center for older adults until she became ill and had to have dialysis three times per week but she remains hopeful that she will return to volunteer, suggesting that she would need to "wait till I get better or something changes." Kat, who previously worked in a factory and later nursing homes, volunteers at the hospital in her community, noting that "it's good to make yourself useful. I give people direction about how to get to places in the hospital." Three of the six women, even when they are ill or have limited financial means to offer others, support their communities with their time and care. For example, the women continue to offer prayers, scripture readings, and counseling to family and community members when they are physically or finanaically unable to contribute.

Transnationalism through the Lens of Critical Race Feminism

On the basis of these counter-stories, I make two separate yet interconnected arguments. The first argues for the importance of financial exchanges between the women and their kinfolk and the second emphasizes the women's familial and community contributions. The connection between the two arguments is the transnational cultural practices that the women assumed while navigating their new country. In other words, they created transnational lives in Canada while maintaining strong and meaningful relationships in the Caribbean. However, Canadian government and white feminist scholars have overlooked the women's resilience, sense of transnational culture, and contributions to the Canadian nation-state. Discussions about Black Caribbean Canadian women often highlight the conditionalities of their immigration to Canada, patterns and experiences of sexist and racist immigration policies, employment discrimination through the West Indian Domestic Scheme, transnational mothering, remittances, and deportation. Consequently, their contributions to Canada are obscured and as Yvonne Bobb-Smith concludes, Caribbean Black women, "particularly in the diaspora of Canada, form a silent majority whose subjugated knowledge and histories of resistance seem never to go beyond their immediate environments" of Caribbean communities abroad (2003, 1).

The findings in this research contradict the majoritarian stories in the media about Caribbean women and older adults. What is clear is that hierarchically, the women have little social power, live in poverty (or would without familial cohabitation), and have various health issues; therefore, their ability to access resources is limited. Nonetheless, in spite the barriers and limitations, the women are generally self-sufficient and not a burden to their families. In addition, this research parallels the extensive information regarding Black women's contribution to building the Canadian nation, and yet their work remains unrecognized in the larger Canadian landscape. This research study explores the women's kin roles and community contributions to make their stories known to a broader audience.

Financial and Physical Well-being

There are two important factors to consider in this discussion: the financial and physical condition of the women. All the women experience poor health with various ailments including heart disease, depression, high blood pressure, and renal failure that requires dialysis. Race, gender, and country of origin influence the women's limited retirement income, but emotional and physical stress from racism is commonly associated with poor health outcomes among Blacks in Canada (James et al. 2010). Activists and scholars note that there is a correlation between poor health and poverty (J. M. Anderson 2000; Dancy and Ralston 2002; Poverty Fact Sheet 2007; Williams and Williams-Morris 2002; Wilson-Ford 1990); therefore, we must link Caribbean Canadian women's health conditions with their financial conditions over their life course. The majoritarian stories suggest that older female Canadians experience poverty because they worked in their homes and did not contribute to the Canada Pension Plan or that they worked in mostly clerical, part-time, and seasonal jobs (Townson 2005). Black

Caribbean Canadian women's counter-stories have a different shape. Utilizing a CRF lens, it is evident that these women continuously worked outside their homes during their productive years. In fact, even though they were more likely to be employed than Canadian-born individuals, they were also more likely to earn less money despite similar qualifications (James 2009; Ornstein 2000; Ornstein and Sharma 1983; Richmond 1993). Most important: counter-stories highlight both the nature of the women's lives and some of the possible reasons for their current health and financial conditions. Critical Race Feminism as a theoretical lens offers a more appropriate position than a gender-based analysis from which to explore and discuss the women's experiences.

I use Critical Race Feminism in this research to recognize the various identity markers that shape women's lives, including race, gender, class, immigrant status, educational level, and marital status—many of these factors place Caribbean Canadian women at the margins of Canadian society. The women's experiences of working in hospitals, factories, nursing homes, and private residences as domestic workers such as nannies, cleaners, and cooks would suggest that gender was the dominant factor in shaping the occupations in which they worked. Attending to a gender-based perspective, a white feminist analysis suggests that women are affected by capitalist patriarchal social arrangements through the sexual division of labor, and that women's experiences in the paid labor market are influenced by their struggle to balance their unpaid domestic responsibilities with their paid employment outside the home (Canadian Women's Foundation 2013; Townson 2000, 2005). Their analysis fails to consider that Black Caribbean Canadian women's paid and unpaid labor occurred simultaneously as they worked as caregivers (e.g., domestic workers and nurses) and that they were deliberately channeled into servitude roles by both Caribbean and Canadian government officials. Furthermore, scholars propose that gender-based discrimination ensures that women traditionally work in the service sector rather than in scientific and technical highly skilled work areas (Canadian Women's Foundation 2013; Townson 2005). Caribbean Canadian women were educated and skilled and yet in some cases they still ended up in unskilled or the lower areas of their professions. This has an impact on the women's income in retirement. Carl E. James notes:

> African Caribbeans, compared to their counterparts with postsecondary education, were more likely—14 percent compared to 9 percent—to obtain their income from government sources. In general, they earned $3,000 less than the average Canadian. But this income differential was significantly less ($5,000) for those African Caribbeans with postsecondary education compared to their counterparts with similar levels of education. This earning differential suggests that the economic return on

education for African-Caribbean Canadians is considerably less than it is for other Canadians. (2009, 99)

Norene Pupo and Ann Duffy (2003) use a majoritarian story to argue that Canada has enshrined women's rights in the Canadian Charter of Rights and Freedoms but, in actuality, government policies reinforce gender bias and discrimination. More specifically, the majoritarian story suggests that women's contribution in the private domestic sphere as caregivers and domestic workers is not recognized in the calculation of Canada Pension Plan payments. This may be the case for white women who stayed home to care for their children. But Black Caribbean Canadian women worked to take care of white Canadians, young and old, and this paid work is not considered real work, so it is not included in the Canadian pension scheme calculations. So although the omission of domestic work as unpaid labor may be correct for some women, this analysis renders older Caribbean Canadian women's paid and unpaid domestic work invisible. Patricia Monture captures this sentiment in her contention that "knowledge is always gendered and raced (although the race is often e-raced)" (2010, x). This research supports other arguments (Beckles 1988; Brand 1988; Safa 1995) and contradicts the notion that men are the primary income earners and therefore heads of households. The arguments of Pupo and Duffy (2003) and the Canadian Women's Foundation (2013) are examples of how "mainstream feminism has paid insufficient attention to the central role of white supremacy subordination of women of color, effectuated by both white men and women" (Wing 2003, 7).

As demonstrated by the participants in this study, Black Caribbean women have always worked inside and outside of the home. Furthermore, Caribbean women have toiled in the fields beside their male counterparts during the brutal transatlantic slavery system (Safa 1995). In the African diaspora, they have always had to work outside the home to support their families or assist their male partners, who are subjected to employment discrimination that negatively affects their ability to provide for their families in the ways white men are afforded (see Beckles and Sheppard 1993, James 2009; Ornstein and Sharma 1983; Richmond 1993; Richmond and Bali 1989). Appropriately, Dionne Brand articulates many Black women's positions when she reminds us that as "class informs our lives, so racism too is an historical determinant in our lives. For us, the relevance of any socio-political theory and of feminist theory especially, depends on its understanding of the role of slavery, of colonialism, and of their attendant racist culture in the development of capitalism" (1987, 28). Indeed, this argument highlights the complexities of Black Caribbean Canadian women's lives on the race, gender, class, and immigrant status axes. It provides a context that helps us to understand why these women are as poor and as sick as they are despite working all their lives to support individuals and institutions transnationally.

Contributions to Family and Community

This research explores older Caribbean Canadian women's contribution beyond their immediate environments and demonstrates their familial and community contributions. Caribbean Canadian women continue to contribute transnationally to their kinfolk in the Caribbean; for some of the women this long-term caring has spanned over forty years. These women send remittances to their families in the Caribbean throughout their life course. Now in their retirement, they are not expected to financially support kinfolk; however, some continue to send remittances to help grandchildren with school-related costs. This commitment to caring for relatives, even after their children are no longer with them, speaks to a level of commitment to family that is not often discussed and therefore not recognized.

Yvonne Bobb-Smith challenges white Canadian sentiments that stereotype Caribbean Canadian women as always being "immigrant women" (2003, 1) regardless of their status, length of time in Canada and social contributions. The findings in this study also contradict this racist and exclusionary notion, which deliberately places these women in the category of Other representing those without connections and belonging to Canada. The women have historically contributed to their communities and families in the Caribbean. I clearly establish here that they contribute similarly to families and communities in Canada.

The women are strong in their faith; they attend church services at least twice per week but they also contribute to the church by paying tithes, giving love offerings, and taking leadership roles in the choir and as prayer mothers. This finding coincides with research suggesting that established immigrants contribute more to their religion organizations than Canadian-born individuals (Scott, Selbee, and Reed 2005). The women minister spiritually to individuals in prison and nursing homes. The importance of religion and spirituality continues as the women age. Elaine A. Brown-Spencer (2006, 2009) and Frances Henry (1994) assert that Caribbeans in Canada experienced racism and exclusion in white church communities as they attempted to adapt to Canadian life and needed to find and create places of worship where they were comfortable. Brand (1991) records that one of the women in her book, Marjorie Lewsey, recalls her mother telling her that most of the Black Caribbeans who lived in Toronto in the early 1920s had to find a Black church when the minister at a prominent white-dominated church told them that they were not welcome in the church. The churches that the Caribbean Canadians formed "became a community infrastructure which responded to the needs of Caribbeans of the Diaspora" (Brown-Spencer 2009) and which continue as a central element in their lives in retirement.

The findings show that older Caribbean Canadian women actively participate in their communities, and they volunteer in various community-based and larger government institutions. Katherine Scott, Kevin Selbee, and Paul Reed (2005) report that immigrants contribute significantly to their communities through volunteering at religious, social services, and sporting organizations, among others. However, the studies do not specifically identify Caribbean Canadian women and Black Canadians, and by extension, Caribbeans are not the faces that are seen in the voluntary discourse. Therefore, this finding about Caribbean Canadian women's voluntary activities is new information. More important: this is an indication that Caribbean women have and continue to contribute to the building and maintenance of the Canadian state in spite of majoritarian stories that suggest otherwise.

Conclusion

Four important themes emerged from this research: (1) the older women continue to send remittances to their families back home; (2) they continue with mothering responsibilities by parenting their grandchildren; (3) they use religious and church affiliations to support members of their Black communities and (4) they contribute to their larger communities through volunteering. These findings have social and health-care implications. Specifically, they can potentially inform policy and program development and implementation in order to provide equitable services to older Caribbean Canadian women. Caribbean Canadian women have aged in place while building the Canadian nation-state and providing kin work transnationally. They supported the building of both nations and families transnationally, and ironically as retirees they continue to give in spite of poor health and poverty. Tragically, neither Canada nor their birth countries have infrastructures to care adequately for them, in part because of majoritarian stories in Canada and lack of finances in the Caribbean and the expectation that families are responsible for caring for older adults. The push factors that dislodged them from their homes and brought them to Canada have worsened and their dreams of returning to the Caribbean to live healthy rich lives require financial resources, in the same way that a "cow kin waan wata," or a cow's skin needs water, in preparation for cooking it for soups and stews.[3] Both Canada and Caribbean countries are implicated in exploiting the women; their governments encourage transnationality while placing the responsibility on vulnerable and already marginalized individuals need to be held accountable to support the people on whose backs the countries are built and maintained.

Older Black Caribbean Canadian women are resilient; they have unique racial and cultural experiences including transnational histories. They left families behind, endured loneliness and harsh social adaptation, rebuilt families, formed organizations, and supported their communities transnationally. In old age, they continue to give both to families in Canada and back home and the wider Canadian communities. We must reciprocate by giving back to them also.

NOTES

1. Canada Pension Plan (CPP)/Quebec Pension Plan (QPP), Old Age Security (OAS), and Guaranteed Income Supplement (GIS) make up Canada's retirement income system. All these benefits can be accessed generally after an individual reaches the age of sixty-five. Canadian citizens and permanent residents are eligible for CPP if they have worked in Canada. The amount is based on the earned wages and the length of time the individual worked. Canadian residents receive OAS regardless of formal work history; and GIS is an income supplement offered to older adults who receive both CPP and OAS and whose monthly income falls below a designated amount (Government of Canada 2015). Retrieved from http://www.servicecanada.gc.ca/eng/audiences/seniors/index.shtml.
2. This is a hissing and/or sucking sound that Caribbean people make by combining movements of their tongues against the side or front teeth. The volume and length of the sound varies depending on the motivation for the action. It is used to express various emotions such as frustration, defiance, anger, irritation, resolution, and sadness. Kissing teeth is not disrespectful but it can be, again depending on how it is applied and in what circumstance (Figueroa and Patrick 2002). In this case, the kiss teeth was meant to emphasize the joy of finding good deals.
3. In the Caribbean all edible parts of animals are used when they are butchered. After the cow is butchered, the skin is taken off in large pieces and subsequently cut in smaller pieces. The hair of the cow is singed off over open fire, scrapped, cut in smaller pieces, washed, and cooked. Cooking the cow's skin can take a few hours and several gallons of water before it is considered soft enough to be consumed.

9

The Recognition and Denial of Kin Work in Palliative Care

Epitomizing Narratives of Canadian Ismaili Muslims

PARIN DOSSA

In this book we have given central space to kin work performed by older persons to recognize and acknowledge their multifaceted contributions transnationally. Here, I argue that dying and death constitute a reflexive moment when one's lifetime work performed in different contexts and sociocultural and political settings is remembered. At the same time, I show that acknowledging the kin work of people at the moment of death is complicated as it is recalled in fragments through conversations, stories, memory work, body language, and sociocultural and religious practices.

An invitation by the British Columbia Hospice Palliative Care Association (BCHPCA) to participate in a panel on Islam and its culture motivated me to explore the relationship between kin work and palliative care. My exposure to medical anthropology had alerted me not to focus exclusively on cultural competence often deployed for the purpose of diagnoses. Aihwa Ong puts it this way, "The health-givers as much as the patients are caught up in the regulatory effects of biomedicine, and cultural material are appropriated only to be incorporated within the medical framework" (1995, 1249). My goal in this chapter is to complicate our understanding of cultural competence by showing that it is more than a mere acknowledgment of values and practices. Ethnographic research lends itself to this task. Its close attention to the minute details of life, its mode of participant observation, and its capacity to open space for participants to tell their stories across sociocultural and political boundaries is enabling. My conversations with my interlocutors from the Ismaili Muslim families did not begin at the time when palliative care was utilized. I came to know the families during the course of my previous research (1985, 1995, and 2009). Knowing the families outside a medicalized unit and over a long period of time is significant, as kin work is a lifetime undertaking, brought into sharp relief at the anticipation of death.

Like many of my participants, I came to Canada as a refugee from Uganda where South Asian communities including Ismaili Muslims had resided for three generations. Ismaili Muslims from Uganda as well as the neighboring countries of Tanzania and Kenya formed my research constituency. In the post-independent period in these East African countries, their status was problematized under the rubric of the Asian Question.[1] Not knowing what the future held for them, many Ismailis and other Asians left the three countries beginning in the early 1970s and settled primarily in Canada, the United States, and England. Contacts were established through BCHPCA, palliative care organizations and their professionals, and during community events that my research assistants and I attended on a regular basis. Our research has taken the form of a multisited ethnography as we engaged with participants at places of their choice: palliative care facilities, public spaces such as cafeterias and community gatherings, and homes. Drawing upon insights from the works of Veena Das (2007), Didier Fassin (2007), and my own earlier work (Dossa 2004), I use the framework of "epitomizing narratives" to analyze the data collected from my longstanding research with the community and more specifically over one year on palliative care (2014–2015).

Epitomizing Narratives

The construct, epitomizing narratives, captures the workings of structural forces as these come to light through singular stories and ethnographic case studies. As such, like the counter-stories described by Delores Mullings (this volume), this construct makes palpable the quotidian and lived realities of people. Such a focus, as Fassin (2007) has argued, enables advocacy and engaged anthropology necessary in a world where social inequality and injustice are the order of the day. In this vein, Das (2007) notes that epitomizing narratives render visible forms of suffering and violence that are otherwise entangled in the inner recesses of life. However, suffering does not go unchallenged as people engage in the task of remaking and reconstructing their lives. These insights have helped me to identify three themes from my data. The first theme identifies the ways that older immigrants accommodate to the busyness of their children and grandchildren through kin work. The second theme discusses how photographs and the conversations over photographs allow for partial recognition of kin work. The third theme illustrates attempts to recreate the aesthetics of home in palliative care centers.

Elders' Kin Work: An Accommodation to the Busyness of Everyday life

Nobody can get beyond everyday life, which literally internalizes global capital-ism, just as global capitalism is nothing without many everyday lives (Merrifield 2006, 10; see Conlon 2011). The processes we are labeling transnational and global are not only produced through the kinds of macro forces that are receiv-ing so much scholarly attention today. They are also crucially produced and experienced through "*the daily life practices and intimate relationships of particular people* as they address questions such as how to age meaningfully in lives that span national-cultural worlds" (Lamb 2007, 133; emphasis added).

The minutiae of everyday life as it unfolds through material objects and sociocultural practices (Conlon 2011), domesticity (Warin and Dennis 2008), discourse (Das 2007), space (Angus et al. 2005), and in the inner recesses of life (Dossa 2014) reveal fractures and ambiguities brought about by structural forces. For example, a focus on everyday life reveals that upon migration, aging women (and men) experience isolation due to the dispersal of families and the busyness of their lives. "Here [in this country], our children do not have time for us. They work and they have children. How much can they do? We tell our children to visit when they can." Sixty-two-year-old Gulshan stated that part of the reason why she tries to be healthy—through walking, good nutrition, and physical exercises—is "because our children will not be able to take care of us if we fall sick." Commenting on how things have changed, Anar noted: "At home [country of birth], if a person passed away she would be remembered as some-one's aunt or cousin or sister, or daughter, or mother or wife. People knew who these kin were and how close or distant were their relationships. People were remembered by their actions and as persons related to other people. Here, it is different. Your kin is not around. Everyone is dispersed. You have to learn to fend for yourself." In sum, older persons find themselves in a different social world where the physical presence of kith and kin is minimal.

A closer reading suggests a politicized script. The busyness of the adult chil-dren is attributed to the pressures placed on immigrants to work hard in a com-petitive neoliberal capitalistic world with its emphasis on individualism and self-responsibility. Furthermore, there is pressure placed on children to do well not only in school, but also in extracurricular activities for which parents give time and invest resources "to give our children the best education so that they can work in any part of the world," as Karim noted. The so-called best education is secular and acquired in Western universities as these have global status and recognition compared with universities in the Global South (see Coe and Shani 2015).[2] The acquisition of higher education is not without a price. Succeeding in a market-oriented world with its emphasis on individualism means spend-ing less time with family. Limited familial time translates into paying greater attention to the future generation than to the previous one. Older migrants are keenly aware of the dilemmas that their own children face in their everyday lives. Consider some of the questions brought to my attention, "Do I take my children for skiing lessons on Sundays or do I take them to my aging parents? Do I take them for music lessons in the evenings or do I send them to a religious night school?" Although some parents sought a balance, older persons nevertheless are keenly aware of the fact that it is the age of youth (*juwaniyano jamano che*). Rather than thinking of themselves, their main concern is that there is not much room left to impart indigenous traditions to the younger generation.

My conversations with older people revealed that they were quick to capture the seriousness of this situation, especially brought about by the loss of the indigenous language of Gujarati. Though this trend began in their East African homelands, it has been accentuated in a new country where the pressure to assimilate and succeed in the market world is strong. Realizing that their own children are busy, older people have taken it upon themselves to "educate" their grandchildren in whatever way they can. Their efforts are not always recognized. This point was brought home to me through the following example.

Accompanied by her mother, fourteen-year-old Salima had brought her ninety-year-old grandmother Kulsum to Jamat Khana (Ismaili mosque referred to as Khane in everyday context). Kulsum was not feeling well. She wanted to leave early while the ceremonies were in progress. Salima informed her mother, who told her to bring her to the drop-off automobile area outside the Jamat Khana. The problem Salima faced was how to get the shoes normally removed by participants when entering the prayer space. Salima went to the shoe area and picked up her shoes as well as those of Kulsum. She went to the drop-off area and left her own shoes outside. She brought Kulsum's shoes inside the prayer space. She helped Kulsum to put on her shoes and guided her to the drop-off area. She realized that the norm of not wearing the shoes did not apply to an old person who could barely walk. But Salima was careful not to put on her own shoes until she was outside the premises of the prayer hall. This seems like a simple example but it is quite intricate. Salima had to use her judgment to not put on her own shoes while ensuring that her grandmother wore her shoes to allow her to use her walker.

Having witnessed this scene, I asked Salima's mother how Salima knew to leave her shoes outside and bring her grandmother her shoes inside in the sacred space. I did not want to dismiss this as common sense. Salima could have worn her shoes along with her grandmother, but instead she signaled her respect for the sacred space by not doing so. Her mother simply stated, "Her grandmother has taught her these things." I did not think much of this incident until I learned about the standing instructions of grandmothers to their grandchildren, "Do not ever forget to say your prayers wherever you are even if this is for two minutes. You have to remember Allah." Reciting prayers for two minutes meant taking the time from secular activities and creating a sacred space momentarily. According to the mothers I talked to, the grandchildren benefited from this practice whether they were writing exams or performing routine work. The grandmothers had shared their own stories of how prayers had helped them during times of crisis and in their everyday lives. Of interest is the fact that the prayers were performed not at the prescribed times (early mornings and evenings) but in the midst of secular activities. Grandparents were mindful of the new and challenging environment where this practice would take place. It is in this context that we can understand how the kin work of older people extended into the wider world rather than remain confined to the discrete space of the home.

Consider another example of a grandmother named Khairoun who resides with her son and his family. Khairoun lights incense and sits on the sofa in the family room at 7:00 A.M. every day without fail. She calls her family members stating that it is *du'a* (prayer) time. She takes a rosary from a glass dish containing several that she has collected for the family. She waits for ten minutes for family members to join her, leaving the decision to them. Those who participate sit cross-legged on the floor. The ten-minute du'a entails rhythmic movements of the body in tune with the recitation of Quranic *ayats* (verses).

Khairoun acknowledged that her three grandchildren and her son and daughter-in-law are busy. "They have to work and the grandchildren are under a lot of pressure at school because of the emphasis on doing very well. They cannot go to Jamat Khana regularly. In my own small way, I would like to remind them of the importance of prayers to be performed every day (*haroz*). And this is why I say my prayers in the living room." Once again, Khairoun's performance of prayer cannot be dismissed as an act that occurs within the private space of a home. When her grandchildren have exams, she advises them to pray because she believes it has a calming effect. She often tells them, "We do our best. Not everything is in our hands. We have to trust in Allah." Though one cannot know for sure, the older women believed that this generational guidance would have its effect. Seventy-two-year-old Fatma put it this way, "If not today, then tomorrow [*ajeh nahi toh kaleh*] they will remember. Today's world is very bad [*bahu kharab jamano che*]. Our children will need faith. Otherwise they will be lost." These observations reveal older generation's keen awareness of the transnational capitalistic world that they perceive in terms of their children's and grandchildren's busyness.

What happens to kin work in palliative care? To being with, I would like to emphasize that the recipients of palliative care are embodied beings who have had a life outside this realm. Older migrants' lived lives encompass border-crossing experiences and are grounded in two or more social worlds. These experiences, I argue, do not come to an end upon the receipt of a terminal diagnoses.

Kin work continues within the unit of palliative care. But it remains unrecognized and may remain in the shadows. An empathetic approach does not, as a matter of fact, include trajectories of transnational lives. The end of life is an opportune moment for one's lifetime work to be recognized and acknowledged.

Meet seventy-one-year-old Shirin and her daughter Noori. I saw them several times at community gatherings. Once they were leaving early and as we live in the same area, I took a ride with them. As we drove, I learnt that Shirin had terminal cancer. Both the mother and the daughter agreed to talk to me upon learning of my project. Noori stated, "Share my mother's story with others. I want people to know about her *seva* [service] and *himat* [courage]." Shirin migrated to Canada in 1976. Given the uncertainty of the political situation in post-independent Kenya, she and her husband left their country of birth with their three children and made Canada their home. The struggles that new immigrants are subject to formed part of their experience. To begin with, the couple's credentials were not recognized. "I had fifteen years of teaching experience. My husband was an accountant back at home. We were told to go back to school to upgrade our qualifications. How can this be possible? We had to educate our children and settle down. I eventually found work as a caregiver and my husband took up sales work." It was a struggle that has not spared their children. Shirin observed, "When my children were in school, they had homework and other activities. When they started work, they were busy building careers. Now they are married they have their own lives. I only ask them to help me if I cannot manage." She recalled an incident whereby she climbed on a stool to get a jar from the top kitchen shelf. She fell down and got hurt. "I did not call my daughter because she was studying." Shirin continued, "We came to this country. We worked hard. I took an early retirement. My work as a caregiver was exhausting. There was a strict care program that we had to follow. It was all rules. There was little time for interaction with the residents. *They [the system] did not understand that caregiving work must include time for social interactions.* How can you do care work and not talk to the residents?" (emphasis added).

Upon retirement, Shirin decided to do voluntary work (seva/service) with seniors in her community. She said that she wanted to fill the gap that she had observed in her workplace—the gap that made her work unrewarding and exhausting. She organized Jamat Khana rides for older congregants. Many use the community buses as their children cannot take them to Khane every day. In Shirin's words,

> They [the children] have busy lives. My job is to see that the drivers (also voluntary) are available. If one is not available, I arrange for another driver from a list that I have. I phone those who are taking the rides and ask them to stay near the door to save time. When Khane is over, I

remind the riders about the bus. I find this work very satisfying. Because of this work, people phone me either to arrange rides or cancel them. This way I get to know them and their problems in life. They talk to me about so many things.

Shirin relayed that her work (seva) for the community gave meaning to her life. In the daytime, she ground spices, ginger, and garlic for her children to save them time. She and her husband also helped with babysitting when required.

Just when she was beginning to feel settled after "many years of hard work," she was diagnosed with terminal cancer.

> It was cancer of the stomach. The doctor said he could not do much for me. He told my daughter Noori that he could refer me for palliative care. I learnt about this form of care from my daughter. The doctor just said it was a better form of care. They would manage my pain and I would be comfortable. Noori decided not to send me to palliative care [in a facility]. She told me if I went and stayed at this place, I would not be able to do my Khane seva. She said, "If doctors take over my care, it would be difficult to ask them if she could take me to *Khane* to do my seva on days when I am better."

In the course of a conversation, I presented Shirin's case to a palliative care nurse. She informed me that they would have accommodated Shirin's desire to continue with her community service provided the doctor gave permission. Shriin and Noori did not raise the issue, assuming that they would be seen as too "demanding." They did not know if they would be granted permission. Their silence was structural. *It was not a matter of language or not knowing what to say but rather that their social positioning as immigrants made them compliant.* They thought that they would be perceived as too demanding and ungrateful if they made a special request.

This point was brought home to me when one of my participants (a care recipient) drank the milk given to her very quickly. When I asked why she drank it so fast, she said: "I do not want to take up the nurse's time. If I drank slowly, she would have to wait to pick up the glass." Shirin and Noori both thought that the doctor would not *understand* why the mother wanted to continue doing community work when she should be taking care of her own health. Shirin was not interested in an individualized form of care, but rather valued social relationships that provided her with a sense of continuity. The difference is significant. As a person taking care of herself she would be a patient. Her personhood, on the other hand, would be affirmed if she was part of the world of social relationships that she had nurtured.

Noori's decision not to send her mother to a palliative care facility to enable her to continue with her service work was not unproblematic. Noori left her job to take care of her mother. She had a palliative nurse come in two hours a day—a service that she discovered later on through a friend. Noori said, "Nobody told us in the beginning that palliative service can take place in our home. I found out after three months." She continued, "My mother is feeling very uncomfortable. She is not used to receiving care from me. She feels guilty that I am not working because of her. I cannot leave her alone during her last days." There is more to a person than being a mere recipient of care and this "more" requires acknowledgment that a person has a history and a life trajectory that needs to be responded to.

Remembering Complex Lives: Family Photographs

It is 4:00 P.M. on a fine day in May 2013. Ashraf suggested that this would be a good time to visit her frail father Sadru whom I had known years ago in Kampala, the city of my birth. As I entered the room in the palliative care facility, she was holding a family photo album. She was showing some pictures to Sadru, recalling old times. One picture was that of the family having a picnic in Entebbe, a popular spot that families visited during weekends. Entebbe is twenty-one miles from Kampala. Other than being the site of an airport, it has beautiful gardens. In the photograph, the family is seated on mats and is enjoying an Asian meal. What is striking about the picture is the get-together of the extended family of aunts, uncles, cousins, siblings, and their children. In the course of viewing the picture, Sadru pointed to a couple of people, describing those who had passed away and those who had dispersed to constitute the family diaspora. In the process, he constructed his own history of migration first to England, then to Toronto, and finally to Vancouver. Each of these movements evoked the presence of the kin that he said was reassuring in his attempt to make a new home.

This encounter triggered my interest in viewing family photographs to explore the kin work of older migrants. This visual genre is unobtrusive as participants tell their own stories through pictures they have taken over the course of their lives. Of interest is the way in which photographs evoke memories of lived lives. Loretta Baldassar (this volume) makes a case for the significance of images and text which can be stored and reflected on. Recall of memory is never for its own sake. Memories are politicized. The past is remembered as a critique of the present; it can speak to and invoke structural forces. Recalling memories through photographs generates a text that is otherwise not articulated. It must be satisfying for Sadru to see the picture of his kin at the moment of death. It would not be an exaggeration to state that a person is validated not as an individual, but rather through a world of social relationships. Second, his construction of a genealogical biography is a means through which he imparts familial knowledge to his children, who otherwise would not have known the kin in the picture due to migration and the dispersal of the family. As his daughter Ashraf noted, "It is because of what my father has told us that I know of all these relatives and the role they played in our lives. My aunty used to send me clothes from Kenya. I never met her. My father told me about his sister [the aunt], their growing up together back at home and her marriage to someone in Kenya. Through him I can imagine what his place of birth was like. I was born in England." Her imagining of life in the diaspora, including the original homeland expands the horizons of her understanding of life and worldview. This understanding of a home away from home is crucial in a globalized world where the boundaries of the nation-state are increasingly becoming fluid and unstable. Here, kin work is significant not only practically, as in Shirin's organization of transportation, but also in terms of generational legacies, as Kristin Elizabeth Yarris in this volume has also noted, including knowledge of diasporic networks.

Although the above scene took place in the supposedly private room of a palliative care facility, it is not exclusively private. Frontline workers enter the room to deliver meals or medication. It is during these *moments* that there is some exchange of information. For example, in the course of photo viewing, a worker may be included momentarily. "You want to see this picture of my father. This picture was taken in Kenya in a small village where he had set up a small shop." Alternatively, the worker might catch snapshots through conversations or pictures. This has also been my experience.

In the course of my interviews with the frontline provider, I raised the following question: "Were there any means through which you came to know the patient beyond your assigned everyday routine of providing meals and taking care of personal hygiene?" In the words of a provider, "It was in the course of serving meals that I learnt a little bit about the lives of my patients. For example one patient did not want to die until he had seen his sister who was going to travel from England. He held on until he had seen her. While he was waiting for her, he told me a little bit about the close ties that the siblings enjoyed as their mother had passed away when they were young."

The worker was touched as his story echoed the loss of her own mother when she was young. A second worker relayed the guilt that her patient felt as he had not patched up his quarrel with his older brother who passed away a couple of months ago. She noted, "When we hear such stories we realize that this is part of being human. This is what our lives are made of." A third worker noted that she had learned how important it was for Muslims to bury a body within twenty-four hours. Her patient's body was not buried for three days as the family was waiting for his two sons to come from England and Kenya respectively. She realized as a result that cultures are not rigid and that "people have global lives." She continued, "The patient I was caring for had global connections. I did not ask him questions about the pictures he showed me about his visits to other countries to see his family. There was one picture from Kenya. It seemed to be special. His whole extended family was there. I felt so sad. Here, he was dying alone. His wife had died. His family was dispersed. I hope I will not be alone when I die."

The point I wish to emphasize is that kin work is activated in palliative care. Recognizing other people's personhood requires acknowledgment of their kin work performed over a lifetime, in sociocultural and also transnational settings. The memorialization of deceased relatives through photos is significant because their kin work is often overlooked. In response to my question to Shamim on how her mother-in-law wanted to be remembered, she said, "No one really knows about her lifetime suffering as a young widow raising five children. She stitched clothes and raised her children. Who will remember her sitting in front of the sewing machine for long hours, *rath ane diwas* [day and night], so that she can educate her children?" Ironically, achievement of high education is the very thing that took her children to far-away places for better economic opportunities. Kin work then is not an idealistic venture. It embodies and reflects ironies and ambiguities of the market-oriented world.

The end of life or the nearness of death is not severed from a life spanning sociocultural and geographical boundaries. A care provider by the name of Manjeet informed me that she held the hand of one woman whom she felt was not going to live for long. Clinging tightly to her hand, the woman told her, "I am not afraid of dying. I wonder how this will happen. How will I go?" Manjeet's response was, "I do not know either. I will learn from you. Let us go through this together." Manjeet was privy to part of the woman's story through a photograph. Photographs and visual memory play an important role in generating such moments. A context-based understanding of one's life can go a long way in creating space for such encounters. It is in this context that I discuss the third theme: The politics of homemaking.

The Politics of Homemaking in an Institutional Environment

An important project for transmigrants is to recreate a sense of home. The home they seek to construct is complicated as they try to include elements from their homeland and those from their new environment. The complication is accentuated by the politics of exclusion that immigrants are subject to. On a general note, Jan Angus and her colleagues have observed, "The sensual experiences of home include odours, food, sounds, decorative touches and use of colour. These sensory, corporeally relevant details are central to comfort, but also constitute the habitual features that allows one to feel 'at home'" (2005, 169). Other than embodying memories of lived life, older migrants keep alive history through material objects such as embroidery, pictures, and other household items. Questions that require consideration are: What happens in a situation where one is compelled to leave one's homeland because of violence and displacement increasingly the case in today's world of global capitalism? What happens when upon migration, older migrants are compelled to leave their homes and move into a nursing home or palliative care facility? The politics of aesthetics come into play when a person's attempt to create a sense of home is compromised because of the workings of the larger system.

Given its philosophy of compassion and care, palliative care facilities create space for families to feel at home. Allowances are made for family members to cook, bring pictures, play music, and bring items of their choice. There is also spatial accommodation as extra beds and showers may be available for family members. However, there is discrepancy between the system and the family's attempt to create a home as illustrated in the following case study of Shamsu and Khamisa.

I met Khamisa in Jamat Khana in February 2009. She and her husband Shamsu had just returned from a trip to India. This was their first visit since their ancestors left this country for East Africa in the early part of the twentieth century. Khamisa invited me to her house to view slides when she learned that I was planning to visit India for the first time. I was struck by the large number of DVDs neatly piled in a corner. Shamsu explained that this was his lifetime work. He was very fond of classical Indian music. He also has a good voice. Khamisa stated that he made tapes of *ginan*, or religious melodies containing meditative knowledge, that he distributed to the children so that they would learn of their tradition. As it is customary to serve tea and snacks [*chai-nasto*], we had *pakodas* made from chickpea flour along with chai. Little did I know that both the DVDs and the pakodas would also reappear in a palliative care facility.

An enduring sense of not feeling well [*takat nathi*] prompted Shamus to seek medical help. Three months went by before Shamsu was diagnosed with terminal cancer. He had leukemia, a condition that he and his wife were familiar with as one of their close friends had died from this disease. According to Khamisa, the doctor was sympathetic but did not provide details. He told them: "There is not much I can do. I will give you referral to a palliative care facility close to your home. You will be well looked after." Not knowing what palliative care was, the couple asked their eldest son to explore this further. The physician informed him that his father had less than six months to live. Khamisa did not go along with this timeline. "There is always hope [*umid*]. In my mind, I did not accept that my husband was going to die. How can this happen? He was not too old [he was seventy-two years old]. He had worked hard all his life. He cannot die so suddenly. It is in Allah's hands."

Khamisa relayed her husband's life narrative in bits and pieces over the course of several weeks. He was born in Dodoma, Tanzania, to a large family of four brothers and two sisters. He started working at the age of fourteen to assist his father in educating his younger siblings. He married Khamisa when he was twenty years old. The precarious situation of South Asians in Tanzania made the family migrate to Canada in the late 1970s. This was the time when Asian properties were nationalized in Tanzania. Like their compatriots, Shamsu and Khamisa went through what has come to be known as the immigrant struggle. This amounts to securing shelter and livelihood at the cost of downward labor-market mobility. It also means working hard for long hours while raising a young family; in their case, a son and a daughter. After a long struggle, the couple bought a house in 1995. "We got our own house and we furnished it according to my husband's wish: leather sofas, mahogany furniture, and a stereo system." The latter was given priority. Khamisa related, "Shamsu loved classical songs. He also sang ginans. When he retired five years ago he spent his time making ginan DVDs that he distributed to family members and friends. He said, 'Let your children learn the ginans. This is the best way to understand our faith and our tradition.' When I go to Khane people remember him. They say, 'Our children learned the ginans through his tapes.'" Six weeks after he was admitted to the palliative care facility, Shamsu passed away at 4:00 A.M., an auspicious moment as congregational prayers are recited at this time. Khamisa noted, "It was not the doctors who decided when he would die. The decision was ultimately made by Allah."

During the time when Shamsu was in the care facility, his wife moved in with him. She slept in the extra bed that was in the room. She only went home to shower and prepare Shamsu's favorite Indian snack—pakodas. Knowing that he always liked to share, she would prepare a large dish. Although Shamsu ate little, he offered the snack to the visitors, maintaining the tradition of hospitality. The aesthetics of serving re-created emotions and feelings. Consumption of food is a social activity. Its sharing in a palliative care unit reverses the exclusive focus on illness, frailty, and death. Shamsu also listened to the DVDs that his brother brought to the facility. While Shamsu's lifetime work of collecting classical Indian songs along with the ginans had always been appreciated, it was acknowledged much more explicitly by friends and family on their visits to the palliative care facility.

Shamsu's desire to have home food was not unusual. The procurement, preparation, and consumption of food encompass realms that are social, political, cultural, and spiritual. Food constitutes part of our way of life, defining who we are as cultural and spiritual beings. It is no wonder that food has assumed importance for diverse groups of people in care institutions: hospitals, nursing homes, and hospices. Whose food is validated in multicultural societies? In the case of Canada, Anglo-European food enjoys dominant status notwithstanding the appropriation of cuisine from other cultures, as is the case of pasta and pizza. Frontline workers informed me that requests for food not considered Anglo-European were considered "special" and only accommodated if the facilities' budgets were not stretched.

I did not think much of the above observations until one day Khamisa asked me to taste pakodas that she had prepared for Shamsu. She told me that this was his favorite food. It evoked memories of his childhood: his mother frying this snack once a week when he returned from school and his visits to a café with his friends to consume it with Indian spiced tea and tamarind sauce. Whenever he went back home, he would ensure that he had a taste of pakodas from the same café, still run by the owner's sons. I found it odd that Khamisa did not serve me the snack for close to fifteen minutes. When I was about to leave, she said, "Wait for a few minutes. I will give you the snack once the nurse has left. She is about to go." When I inquired further, she said, "I want to warm it up but I do not know if the nurse would like the aroma spreading all over the place." Khamisa's attempt not to give offense to an authority figure in the institution was based on her work experience: "When I went to work, I did not take our food [apnuh khawanu]. This is because when I warmed it up, other women in my office gave me looks. I felt uncomfortable. I only took a sandwich. I did not quite like it but it was better this way." The younger generation I talked to noted that now there is more acceptance of their food in public places.

Khamisa also maintained a low profile when it came to playing the audio tapes that Shamsu enjoyed. At times, she would lower the volume—rendering invisible his legacy of kin work. In the way of explanation she said: "I do not want to disturb anyone. They [the nurses] will think we are not grateful." The message of self-regulation of difference is conveyed to immigrants in strong terms. Otherwise as Sarah Mahler has argued in *American Dreaming*, "If the image associated with immigrants is full of positive qualifiers such as 'hard-working,' 'community-minded,' and mutually supportive [to which I would add 'compliant'], it serves to identify them more strongly with the ideal American temperament" (1995, 227). Otherwise, she continues "a wedge is driven between them and natives." Furthermore, Khamisa is dependent on the nurses' goodwill in caring for her sick husband.

Food and the DVDs that Shamsu collected—his lifetime work—constitute kin work as both nurture sociocultural relationships intergenerationally and create a sense of feeling at home, a premise adopted in palliative care. Doris, a frontline worker observed, "When patients are admitted into hospice, we endeavour to make them feel at home. We try and meet their wishes." In reality, this may not happen. Palliative care—like its parent body, the Canadian health system—has yet to address the concerns and aspirations of racialized minorities (Giesbrecht 2014). And these concerns, I would argue, should include an understanding of the aesthetics of home—including its sound-, smell-, and taste-scapes—which index cherished values and practices from the homeland as well as the country of settlement. When I presented Khamisa's case study to the frontline workers, I received the following responses.

JUDY: It is their private space. We do not interfere. We encourage families to fulfill the wishes of their loved ones provided it is safe and does not create disturbance.

RUTH: I would have loved to ask the family more about *their* food. I am very interested. I am not sure they would have talked to me about *their cultural practices* and their private matters [emphasis in the original].

KELLY: Now that you have shared this example, I will make it a point to take more interest. I think that these situations humanize our patients. And we should take interest.

The above conversations reveal a paradox. There could be room for the public performance of kin work in palliative care, hence creating a feeling and aesthetics of being at home. But this goal is not achieved because of the private/public divide which in actual fact translates into "them" and "us," prevalent in a country where immigrants are the Other (Bannerji 1995, 2000; Razack 1998; Thobani 2007). Public acknowledgment of food and music would have helped Khamisa and her husband feel more at home.

I am not suggesting that palliative care professionals should bear the burden of initiating strategies that may not be practical. The point I want to emphasize is that food is a medium that breaks barriers as much as it can create others. As food features prominently in palliative care settings, greater awareness of this everyday practice can go a long way in recognizing another's humanness.

In my attempt to pursue the question of aesthetics of home and what makes us human, I asked my interlocutors for what it was like to die in their homeland where "palliative care" was not available. Jamila shared the following account with me.

I remember when I was in secondary school my mother took care of my grandmother in Uganda. She was eighty-eight years old. She was sick and bedridden. We all knew that she was not going to live long. My mother said, "Allah will take her, when it is her time to die. It is not in our hands." Her bed was placed in the living room right close to the main entrance. Whoever came to the house whether they were visitors or the children back from school, we would all greet her. How could we miss her? She was right there. We felt her presence. Although she was sick and frail, she was a strong woman. She would talk to us and tell us stories even when she was not well. My mother said: "Seeing people and talking to them lessened her pain." She died peacefully as if she had chosen the time of her death. This was when we had come back from school and we were all present in the room. On the day she died, she had refused to take her medication. She knew that it was her last day and she wanted to be "awake."

As an afterword, Jamila noted: "My grandmother taught us about dying and death." Contrary to our expectation that palliative care is a new phenomenon originating in the West, its deinstitutionalized existence in other cultural traditions requires acknowledgment. In today's world of high technology, what Jamila describes may be considered rudimentary. But this is a misconception. Without romanticizing this form of home-based care, I would like to highlight some of the elements that we may want to revisit: the social visibility of the care recipient as opposed to confinement to a room or a separate facility, the fostering of social relationships through visitors and children, and management of pain to the extent possible through social activity and self-care. In the case of the latter, I learned that the grandmother stretched parts of her body as a form of "exercise" to ease her pain. This is not a typical example and it has shortcomings such as gendered-based care, lack of privacy, and reduced quality of life owing to the unavailability of medication. At the same time, the grandmother's personhood was not diminished. Her physical and social visibility, her ability to share stories, and her control over the moment of death are elements worth noting. The patient-centered focus of palliative care is premised on fulfilling the wishes of the patient as an individual and not as a person embedded in a world of social relationships—the bedrock of kin work.

Conclusion

In this chapter, I have highlighted the significance of kin work in a transnational setting. Taking the example of older Ismaili migrants, I have shown that the acknowledgment of multifaceted kin work can validate the lives of people who are otherwise marginalized. The kin work of aging migrants speak to structural forces, the most salient of which is the busyness of children's lives embedded in a global capitalistic system with its emphasis on individualism and self-responsibility. How can the kin work of older migrants be validated? In response to this question I have adopted two lines of inquiry. The first one concerns shifting what is considered a home-based and therefore "private" performance of kin work into the public space of palliative care, administered institutionally in a hospital or hospice setting or at home. I have shown that older people on their death beds receive the attention of kin who are otherwise busy. I came across several examples of sons or daughters taking a leave of absence to be with their father or mother in the last days of their lives. Family and kin traveling from other places was also a common scenario. Palliative care and the impending arrival of death provided the space for the recognition of kin work.

Second, early in my research I recognized that validating the lives of marginalized populations requires an analytical framework that lends itself to nuanced insights. This is the reason why my usage of the construct of kin work does not merely rest at the level of activities or social relationships. My goal is to use kin work as a construct that recognizes the lives of older migrants at multiple levels, including continuity or disjuncture between here and there (home and host countries) and also at a collective level. Given the commonality of history and trajectory of migration, one person's kin work encapsulates those of his or her cohort. It is for this reason that I framed my analysis within the overarching framework of epitomizing narratives within which I identify three themes suggested by my ethnographic data: (a) everyday life, the significance of which is recognized at multiple levels through which marginalized actors speak to the systems of power; (b) visual memory, the significance of which lies in the reconstruction of lives reaching their final years on this earth; and (c) a politics of aesthetics in reimagining a home through such mediums as food and music. What has been buried—the archeology of knowledge, as Foucault (1972) would put it—can come to light in the form of valued legacies.

Ethnographic research made it possible for me to conduct field work at multiple sites, including the homes of participants, community gatherings, public spaces, especially cafeterias, and, to a limited extent, palliative care facilities. Out of respect for the challenging times that families were faced with, I did not visit the facilities unless I received an invitation to drop in. In some ways this limitation proved to be advantageous as I was compelled to explore storied lives. This context made me realize the expanse of kin work as families recalled the work of their loved ones that might not have otherwise come to light.

Ethnographic research requires that we facilitate conversation between professionals and families and their loved one. The foundation for such a conversation must be the recognition that the person receiving palliative care has lived a life beyond the space of palliative care—a life that has crossed geopolitical and cultural boundaries and a life that has been engaged in doing work (kin work) that speaks to the issues of our times as Sarah Lamb (2009) has so well documented. The palliative care philosophy of compassionate patient-oriented care would be well served if its practitioners take into account the kin work of transnational migrants. Rather than appearing as care recipients of bed and body work, the latter would be seen as persons whose lives embody imprints of their lifetime revealed through kin work.

ACKNOWLEDGMENTS

This chapter is part of a larger project funded by: (a) Small SSHRC Grant, Simon Fraser University and (b) Simon Fraser University: Community Initiative Grant.

NOTES

1. The Asian Question refers to the precarious status in which the Asians were positioned by the British colonial system: below the Europeans and above the indigenous Africans.
2. Using the term "cultural capital," Cati Coe and Serah Shani (2015) capture the dilemmas that immigrant families are confronted with as they seek to impart Western education to their children while ensuring that their cultural values and traditions are maintained.

ACKNOWLEDGMENTS

The genesis of this volume has its origins in the realization that the lives and work of older transnational migrants are not acknowledged. To render visible what has remained in the background, we employ the construct of kin work that include care and service work, market-based contributions, affect, repertoires of knowledge, the sustenance of familial and social ties, and the nurturing of communities. Kin work comes to light at critical moments of migration, border-crossing and resettlement as well as in the context of everyday life in homelands and diasporas. In order to meet our goal of documenting this project, we invited scholars who had undertaken fieldwork on aging and old age in different parts of the world. We are grateful for their contributions to the volume.

We owe a debt of gratitude to all the women and men who participated in this work and brought it to fruition. Sarah Lamb inspired and encouraged us to undertake what proved to be a challenging endeavor. Marlie Wasserman and Kimberly Guinta at Rutgers University Press gave us their guidance, support, and constructive criticism. Two anonymous reviewers gave us excellent feedback on the volume, and their comments were most helpful. It has been a pleasure to work with freelance editor Kate Moreau, Marilyn Campbell, and Carrie Hudak from Rutgers University Press. Thank you all for your support.

Partial funding for the book publication was provided by the University Publication Fund at Simon Fraser University.

REFERENCES

Aboderin, Isabella. 2004. "Decline in Material Family Support for Older People in Urban Ghana, Africa: Understanding Processes and Causes of Change." *Journal of Gerontology* 59B(3): S128–S137.

———. 2006. *Intergenerational Support and Old Age in Africa.* New Brunswick, NJ: Transaction Publishers.

Abrego, Leisy. 2014. *Sacrificing Families: Navigating Laws, Labor, and Love across Borders.* Stanford, CA: Stanford University Press.

Acharya, Manju, and Herbert Northcott. 2007. "Mental Distress and the Coping Strategies of Elderly Indian Immigrant Women." *Transcultural Psychiatry* 44(4): 614–636.

Ackers, Louise. 1998. *Shifting Spaces: Women, Citizenship, and Migration within the European Union.* Bristol, UK: Policy Press.

———. 2004. "Citizenship, Migration, and the Valuation of Care in the European Union." *Journal of Ethnic and Migration Studies* 30(2): 373–396.

Ackers, Louise, and Peter Dwyer. 2002. *Senior Citizenship? Retirement, Migration, and Welfare in the European Union.* Bristol, UK: Policy Press.

Ahmed, Ali M., Lina Andersson, and Mats Hammerstedt. 2012. "Does Age Matter for Employability? A Field Experiment on Ageism in the Swedish Labor Market." *Applied Economics Letters* 19: 403–406.

Albert, Rocío, Lorenzo Escot, and José Andrés Fernández-Cornejo. 2011. "A Field Experiment to Study Sex and Age Discrimination in the Madrid Labor Market." *International Journal of Human Resource Management* 22(2): 351–375.

Allahar, Anton. 2010a. "At Home in the Caribbean Diaspora: 'Race' and the Dialectics of Identity." *Wadabagei* 3(1): 2–28.

———. 2010b. "The Political Economy of 'Race' and Class in Canada's Caribbean Diaspora." *American Review of Political Economy* 8(2): 54–86.

Allendorf, Keera. 2013. "Going Nuclear? Family Structure and Women's Health in India, 1996–2006." *Demography* 50(3): 853–880.

Ammann, Eva Soom, and Karin van Holten. 2013. "Getting Old Here and There: Opportunities and Pitfalls of Transnational Care Arrangements." *Transnational Social Review* 3(1): 31–47.

Anagnost, Ann. 1997. "Neo-Malthusian Fantasy and National Transcendence." In *National Past-Times: Narrative, Representation, and Power in Modern China*, edited by Ann Anagnost, 117–137. Durham, NC: Duke University Press.

———. 2004. "The Corporeal Politics of Quality (*Suzhi*)." *Public Culture* 2 (Spring): 189–208.

Andall, Jacqueline. 2000. *Gender, Migration and Domestic Service: The Politics of Black Women in Italy.* Interdisciplinary Research Series in Ethnic, Gender, and Class Relations. Aldershot, UK: Ashgate.

———. 2013. "Gendered Mobilities and Work in Europe: An Introduction." *Journal of Ethnic and Migration Studies* 39(4): 525–534.

Anderson, Bridget. 2000. *Doing the Dirty Work? The Global Politics of Domestic Labor.* New York: Palgrave Macmillan.

Anderson, Joan M. 2000. "Gender, 'Race,' Poverty, Health, and Discourses of Health Reform in the Context of Globalization: A Postcolonial Feminist Perspective in Policy Research." *Nursing Inquiry* 7(4): 220–229.

Angus, Jan, Pia Kontos, Isabel Dyck, Patricia McKeever, and Blake Poland. 2005. "The Personal Significance of Home: Habitus and the Experience of Receiving Long-Term Home Care." *Sociology of Health and Illness* 27(2): 161–187.

Apt, Nana Araba. 1996. *Coping with Old Age in a Changing Africa.* Aldershot, UK: Avebury.

Ariès, Philippe. 1962. *Centuries of Childhood: A Social History of Family Life.* Translated by R. Baldick. New York: Vintage Books.

Armstrong, B., and S. Taylor. 2000. *Tireless Champion of Just Causes: Memoirs of Bromley L. Pickering.* Ontario: Vitabu Publishing.

Aronson, Jane, and Sheila M. Neysmith. 2006. "Obscuring the Costs of Home Care: Restructuring at Work." *Work, Employment, and Society* 20: 27–45.

Atkinson, Rowland, and John Flint. 2001. "Accessing Hidden and Hard-to-Reach Populations: Snowball Research Strategies." *Social Research Update* 33(1): 1–4.

Attride-Stirling, Jennifer. 2001. "Thematic Networks: An Analytic Tool for Qualitative Research." *Qualitative Research* 1(3): 385–405.

Aylward, Carol A. 1999. *Canadian Critical Race Theory: Racisms and the Law.* Halifax: Fernwood.

Baker, Sarah Elsie, and Rosalind Edwards. 2012. "How Many Qualitative Interviews Is Enough? National Centre for Research Methods Review Discussion Paper." Available at http://eprints.ncrm.ac.uk/2273/4/how_many_interviews.pdf, accessed March 1, 2015.

Bakken, Borge. 2000. *The Exemplary Society.* Oxford: Oxford University Press.

Baldassar, Loretta. 2001. *Visits Home: Migration Experiences between Italy and Australia.* Melbourne: Melbourne University Press.

———. 2007. "Transnational Families and the Provision of Moral and Emotional Support: The Relationship between Truth and Distance." *Identities* 14(4): 385–409.

———. 2008. "Missing Kin and Longing to Be Together: Emotions and the Construction of Co-presence in Transnational Relationships." *Journal of Intercultural Studies* 29(3): 247–266.

———. 2014. "Too Sick to Move: Distant 'Crisis' Care in Transnational Families." *International Review of Sociology* 24(3): 391–405.

———. 2015. "Guilty Feelings and the Guilt Trip: Emotions and Motivation in Migration and Transnational Caregiving." *Emotion, Space, and Society* 16: 81–89.

———. 2016a. "De-demonising Distance in Mobile Family Lives: Co-presence, Care Circulation, and Polymedia as Vibrant Matter." *Journal of Global Networks* 16(2): 145–163.

———. 2016b. "Mobilities and Communication Technologies: Transforming Care in Family Life." In *Family Live in an Age of Migration and Mobility: Global Perspectives through the Life Course,* edited by Majella Kilkey and Ewa Palenga-Möllenbeck. New York: Macmillan.

Baldassar, Loretta, Cora Vellekoop Baldock, and Raelene Wilding. 2007. *Families Caring across Borders: Migration, Ageing, and Transnational Caregiving.* Houndmills, UK: Palgrave Macmillan.

Baldassar, Loretta, Majella Kilkey, Laura Merla, and Raelene Wilding. 2014. "Transnational Families." In *The Wiley-Blackwell Companion to the Sociology of Families*, edited by Judith Treas, Jacqueline Scott, and Martin Richards, 155–175. Oxford: John Wiley and Sons.

Baldassar, Loretta, and Laura Merla, eds. 2013. *Transnational Families, Migration, and the Circulation of Care: Understanding Mobility and Absence in Family Life*. London: Routledge.

Baldassar, Loretta, and Joanne Pyke. 2014. "Intra-diaspora Knowledge Transfer and 'New' Italian Migration." *International Migration* 52(4): 128–143.

Baldassar, Loretta, Raelene Whiting, and Cora Baldock. 2007. "Long-Distance Caregiving: Transnational Families and the Provision of Aged Care." In *Family Caregiving for Older Disabled People*, edited by Isabella Paoletti, 201–227. New York: Nova Science.

Baldock, Cora Vellekoop. 2000. "Migrants and Their Parents." *Journal of Family Issues* 21(2): 205–224.

———. 2003. "Long-Distance Migrants and Family Support: A Dutch Case Study." *Health Sociology Review* 12(1): 45–54.

Balgamwalla, Sabrina. 2014. "Bride and Prejudice: How U.S. Immigration Law Discriminates against Spousal Visa Holders." *Berkeley Journal of Gender, Law, and Justice* 29(1): 25–71.

Bannerji, Himani. 1995. *Thinking Through: Essays on Feminism, Marxism, and Anti-Racism*. Toronto: Women's Press.

———. 2000. *The Dark Side of the Nation: Essays on Multiculturalism, Nationalism, and Gender*. Toronto: Canadian Scholars' Press.

Basch, Linda, Nina Glick Schiller, and Christina Szanton Blanc. 2008. "Transnational Projects: A New Perspective and Theoretical Premises." In *The Transnational Studies Reader: Intersections and Innovations*, edited by Sanjeev Khagram and Peggy Levitt, 261–272. New York: Routledge.

Bastia, Tanja. 2009. "Women's Migration and the Crisis of Care: Grandmothers Caring for Grandchildren in Urban Bolivia." *Gender and Development* 17(3): 389–401.

Battams, Nathan. 2013. "In It Together: Multigenerational Living in Canada." *Transition* 43(3): 11–13.

Baykara-Krumme, Helen. 2013. "Returning, Staying, or Both? Mobility Patterns among Elderly Turkish Migrants after Retirement." *Transnational Social Review* 3(1): 11–29.

Beckles, Hilary. 1988. *Afro-Caribbean Women and Resistance to Slavery in Barbados*. London: Karnak House.

———. 1989. *Corporate Power in Barbados: The Mutual Affair: Economic Injustice in a Political Democracy*. Bridgetown, Barbados: Lighthouse Communications.

Beckles, Hilary, and Verene Shepherd. 1993. *Caribbean Freedom: Society and Economy from Emancipation to the Present*. Kingston, Jamaica: James Currey.

Bernhard, Judith K., Patricia Landolt, and Luin Goldring. 2009. "Transnationalizing Families: Canadian Immigration Policy and the Spatial Fragmentation of Care-Giving among Latin American Newcomers." *International Migration* 47(2): 3–31.

Berry, Theodorea Regina. 2009. "Women of Color in a Bilingual/Dialectal Dilemma: Critical Race Feminism against a Curriculum of Oppression in Teacher Education." *International Journal of Qualitative Studies in Education* 22(6): 745–753.

Biehl, João. 2005. *Vita: Life in a Zone of Social Abandonment*. Berkeley: University of California Press.

Black, Helen K. 2000. "Life as Gift: Spiritual Narratives of Elderly African-American Women Living in Poverty." *Journal of Aging Studies* 13(4): 441–455.

Blair, Thomas. 2012. "'Community Ambassadors' for South Asian Elder Immigrants: Late-Life Acculturation and the Roles of Community Health Workers." *Social Science and Medicine* 75(10): 1769–1777.

Bloch, Maurice E. F. 1998. *How We Think They Think: Anthropological Approaches to Cognition, Memory, and Literacy*. Boulder, CO: Westview Press.

Bobb-Smith, Yvonne. 2003. *I Know Who I Am: A Caribbean Woman's Identity in Canada*. Toronto: Women's Press.

Boccagni, Paolo. 2012. "Practising Motherhood at a Distance: Retention and Loss in Ecuadorian Transnational Families." *Journal of Ethnic and Migration Studies* 38(2): 261–277.

Boehm, Deborah A. 2012. *Intimate Migrations: Gender, Family, and Illegality among Transnational Mexicans*. New York: New York University Press.

Boris, Eileen, and Jennifer Klein. 2012. *Caring for America: Home Health Workers in the Shadow of the Welfare State*. New York: Oxford University Press.

Bosworth, Richard. 1988. "Official Italy Rediscovers Australia 1945–1950." *Affari sociali internazionali* 26(2): 59–60.

Boucher, Anna. 2007. "Skill, Migration, and Gender in Australia and Canada: The Case of Gender-Based Analysis." *Australian Journal of Political Science* 42(3): 383–401.

Bourdieu, Pierre. 1977. *Outline of a Theory of Practice*. Translated by Richard Nice. New York: Cambridge University Press.

Brand, Dionne. 1987. "Black Women and Work: The Impact of Racially Constructed Gender Roles on the Sexual Division of Labor." *Fireweed* 25: 28.

———. 1988. "Black Women and Work: The Impact of Racially Constructed Gender Roles on the Sexual Division of Labor; Part Two." *Fireweed* 26: 87.

———. 1991. *No Burden to Carry: Narratives of Black Working Women in Ontario, 1920s–1950s*. Toronto: Women's Press.

Brown-Spencer, Elaine A. 2006. "Spiritual Politics: Politicizing the Black Church Tradition in Anti-Colonial Praxis." In *Anti-Colonialism and Education: The Politics of Resistance*, edited by George J. Sefa Dei and Arlo Kempf, 107–127. Toronto: Sense Publication.

———. 2009. "The Black Oneness Church in Perspective." Ph.D. diss., Ontario Institute for Studies in Education of the University of Toronto. Available at https://tspace.library .utoronto.ca/bitstream/1807/19177/1/brownspencer_elaine_a_200911_phd_thesis.pdf, accessed June 23, 2015.

Bruner, Jerome S. 2003. *Making Stories: Law, Literature, Life*. New York: Farrar, Straus and Giroux.

Bryceson, Deborah Fahy, and Ulla Vuorela, eds. 2002. *The Transnational Family: New European Frontiers and Global Networks*. Cross-Cultural Perspectives on Women. Oxford: Berg.

Brydon, Lynne. 1979. "Women at Work: Some Changes in Family Structure in Amedzofe-Avatime, Ghana." *Africa* 49(2): 97–111.

Bryman, Alan. 2001. *Social Research Methods*. Oxford: Oxford University Press.

Bureau of Labor Statistics. 2013. "Fastest Growing Occupations." Available at http://www.bls .gov/emp/ep_table_103.htm, accessed December 11, 2014. 2014.

———. 2014. "Nursing Assistants and Orderlies." *Occupational Outlook Handbook, 2014–15 Edition*. Available at http://www.bls.gov/ooh/healthcare/nursing-assistants.htm, accessed December 11.

Caldwell, John C. 1969. *African Rural-Urban Migration: The Movement to Ghana's Towns*. Canberra, Australia: Australian National University Press.

Calliste, Agnes. 1989. "Canada's Immigration Policy and Domestics from the Caribbean: The Second Domestic Scheme." *Race, Class, Gender: Bonds and Barriers* 5: 133–165.

———. 1993a. "Race, Gender, and Canadian Immigration Policy: Blacks from the Caribbean, 1900–1932." *Journal of Canadian Studies* 28(4): 131–140.

———. 1993b. "Women of Exceptional Merit: Immigration of Caribbean Nurses to Canada." *Canadian Journal of Women and the Law* 6: 85–103.

Canadian Women's Federation. 2013. "Facts about Women and Poverty." Available at http://www.canadianwomen.org/facts-about-poverty, accessed July 23, 2015.

CBC News. 2014. "Canada Accepting 5,000 Parent, Grandparent Sponsorship Applications." Available at http://www.cbc.ca/news/politics/canada-accepting-5-000-parent-grand parent-sponsorship-applications-1.2481803, accessed January 3, 2015.

Cecil, Robert Gerald, and G. Edward Ebanks. 1992. "The Caribbean Migrant Farm Worker Programme in Ontario: Seasonal Expansion of West Indian Economic Spaces." *International Migration* 30(1): 19–37.

Chamberlain, Mary. 1997. *Narratives of Exile and Return.* London: Macmillan Caribbean.

____. 1998. "Brothers and Sisters, Uncles and Aunts: A Lateral Perspectives on Caribbean Families in Britain." In *The New Family*, edited by Elizabeth Bortolia Silva and Carol Smart, 129–142. London: Sage.

Chappell, Neena, and Margaret Penning. 2009. *Understanding Health, Health Care, and Health Policy in Canada.* Toronto: Oxford University Press.

Chatters, Linda M., Robert Joseph Taylor, James S. Jackson, and Karen D. Lincoln. 2008. "Religious Coping among African Americans, Caribbean Blacks, and Non Hispanic Whites." *Journal of Community Psychology* 36(3): 371–386.

Chatters, Linda M., Robert Joseph Taylor, Karen D. Lincoln, Ann Nguyen, and Sean Joe. 2011. "Church-Based Social Support and Suicidality among African Americans and Black Caribbeans." *Archives of Suicide Research* 15(4): 337–353.

Chaudhuri, Himadri Roy, and Sitanath Majumdar. 2006. "Of Diamonds and Desires: Understanding Conspicuous Consumption from a Contemporary Marketing Perspective." *Academy of Marketing Science Review* 11: 1–18.

Chee, Maria W. L. 2005. *Taiwanese American Transnational Families: Women and Kin Work.* New York: Routledge.

Chen, Feinian, Guangya Lu, and Christine A. Mair. 2011. "Intergenerational Ties in Context: Grandparents Caring for Grandchildren in China." *Social Forces* 90(2): 571–594.

Chen, Feizh. 2006. "Tanqin laoren haiwai zaoyu qinqing taiozhan [Chinese seniors confront challenges in relationship when visiting their families overseas]." *People's Daily* (Oversea Version). Available at http://news.xinhuanet.com/overseas/2006-08/04/content_4916476.htm, accessed July 12, 2011.

Cheung, Chau-Kiu, and Alex Yui-huen Kwan. 2009. "The Erosion of Filial Piety by Modernisation in Chinese Cities." *Ageing and Society* 29(1): 179–198.

Chiang, Nora Lan-Hung. 2008. "'Astronaut Families': Transnational Lives of Middle-Class Taiwanese Married Women in Canada." *Social and Cultural Geography* 9: 505–518.

Chodos, Robert. 1977. *The Caribbean Connection.* Toronto: Lorimer.

Chou, Rita Jing-Ann. 2011. "Filial Piety by Contract? The Emergence, Implementation, and Implications of the 'Family Support Agreement' in China." *Gerontologist* 51(1): 3–16.

Choudhry, Usha. 2001. "Uprooting and Resettlement Experiences of South Asian Immigrant Women." *Western Journal of Nursing Research* 23(4): 376–393.

Choy, Catherine Ceniza. 2003. *Empire of Care: Nursing and Migration in Filipino American History.* Durham, NC: Duke University Press.

Citizenship and Immigration Canada. 2013. "Backgrounder: Action Plan for Faster Family Reunification: Phase II." Available at: http://www.cic.gc.ca/english/department/media/backgrounders/2013/2013-05-10b.asp accessed May 28, 2014.

Clark, Rebecca L., Jennifer E. Glick, and Regina M. Bures. 2009. "Immigrant Families over the Life Course: Research Directions and Needs." *Journal of Family Issues* 30: 852–872.

Clarke, John. 2005. "Welfare States as Nation States: Some Conceptual Reflections." *Social Policy and Society* 4: 407–415.

Cockburn, Patrick J. L. 2013. "Street Papers, Work, and Begging: Experimenting at the Margins of Economic Legitimacy." *Journal of Cultural Economy* 7(2): 145–160.

Coe, Cati. 2011. "What Is Love? The Materiality of Care in Ghanaian Transnational Families." *International Migration* 49(6): 7–24.

——. 2012a. "Growing Up and Going Abroad: How Ghanaian Children Imagine Transnational Migration." *Journal of Ethnic and Migration Studies* 38(6): 913–931.

——. 2012b. "Transnational Parenting: Child Fostering in Ghanaian Immigrant Families." In *Young Children of Black Immigrants in America: Changing Flows, Changing Faces*, edited by Randy Capps and Michael Fix, 265–296. Washington, DC: Migration Policy Institute.

——. 2013. *The Scattered Family: Parenting, African Migrants, and Global Inequality.* Chicago: University of Chicago Press.

——. 2016. "Orchestrating Care in Time: Ghanaian Migrant Women, Family, and Reciprocity." *American Anthropologist* 118(1): 37–48.

Coe, Cati, and Serah Shani. 2015. "Cultural Capital and Transnational Parenting: The Case of Ghanaian Migrants in the United States." *Harvard Education Review* 85(4): 562–586.

Cohen, Lawrence. 1998. *No Aging in India: Alzheimer's, the Bad Family, and Other Modern Things.* Berkeley: University of California Press.

Cohler, Bertram J., and Andrew J. Hostetler. 2003. Linking Life Course and Life Story: Social Change and the Narrative Study of Lives. In *Handbook of the Life Course*, edited by Jeylan T. Mortimer and Michael J. Shanahan, 555–578. New York: Kluwer Academic/Plenum.

Cole, Jennifer. 2007. "Fresh Contact in Tamatave, Madagascar: Sex, Money, and Intergenerational Transformation." In *Generations and Globalization: Youth, Age, and Family in the New World Economy*, edited by Jennifer Cole and Deborah Durham, 74–101. Bloomington: Indiana University Press.

——. 2013. "On Generations and Aging: 'Fresh Contact' of a Different Sort." In *Transitions and Transformations: Cultural Perspectives on Aging and the Life Course*, edited by Caitrin Lynch and Jason Danely, 218–230. New York: Berghahn.

Cole, Jennifer, and Deborah Durham, eds. 2007. *Generations and Globalization: Youth, Age, and Family in the New World Economy.* Bloomington: Indiana University Press.

Collins, Patricia Hill. 1994. "Shifting the Center: Race, Class, and Feminist Theorizing about Motherhood." In *Mothering: Ideology, Experience, and Agency*, edited by Evelyn Nakano Glenn, Grace Change, and Linda Rennie Forcey, 45–65. New York: Routledge.

——. 1997. "The Meaning of Motherhood in Black Culture and Black Mother-Daughter Relationships." In *Toward a New Psychology of Gender*, edited by Mary Gergen and Sara N. Davis, 326–340. New York: Routledge.

Conlon, Deirdre. 2011. "A Fractured Mosaic: Encounters with the Everyday amongst Refugee and Asylum Seeker Women." *Population, Space, and Place* 17: 714–726.

Cook, Sarah, and Xiao yuan Dong. 2011. "Harsh Choices: Chinese Women's Paid Work and Unpaid Care Responsibilities under Economic Reform." *Development and Change* 42(4): 947–65.

Cooper, Afua. 2006. *The Hanging of Angélique: The Untold Story of Canadian Slavery and the Burning of Old Montreal.* Athens: University of Georgia Press.

Coutin, Susan Bibler. 2005. "The Formation and Transformation of Central American Community Organizations in Los Angeles." In *Latino Los Angeles: Transformations, Communities, and Activism*, edited by Gilda Ochoa and Enrique Ochoa, 155–177. Tucson: University of Arizona Press.

Crary, David. 2010. "Adopting China's Special-Needs Kids." *NBCNews.com* March 28. Available at http://www.nbcnews.com/id/36037857/ns/health-childrens_health/t/adopting -chinas-special-needs-kids/#.Ud6xN3asswJ, accessed December 22, 2010.

Crawford, Charmaine. 2003. "Sending Love in a Barrel: The Making of Transnational Caribbean Families in Canada." *Canadian Woman Studies* 22(3): 104–109.

Crenshaw, Kimberlé. 1989. "Demarginalizing the Intersection of Race and Sex: A Black Feminist Critique of Antidiscrimination Doctrine, Feminist Theory, and Antiracist Politics." *University of Chicago Legal Forum* 140: 139–167.

———. 1995. "Race, Reform, and Retrenchment: Transformation and Legitimation in Antidiscrimination Law." In *Critical Race Theory: The Key Writings That Formed the Movement*, edited by Kimberlé Williams, Neil Gotanda, Gary Peller, and Kendall Thomas, 103–122. New York: The New Press.

Crockett, Lisa. 2002. "Agency in the Life Course: Concepts and Processes." *Agency, Motivation, and the Life Course* 48: 1–31.

Croll, Elisabeth J. 2006. "The Intergenerational Contract in the Changing Asian Family." *Oxford Development Studies* 34(4): 473–491.

Cuadraz, Gloria, and Lynet Uttal. 1999. "Intersectionality and In-depth Interviews: Methodological Strategies for Analyzing Race, Class, and Gender." *Race, Gender, Class* 6: 156–181.

Da, Wei Wei. 2003. "Transnational Grandparenting: Child Care Arrangements among Migrants from the People's Republic of China to Australia." *Journal of International Migration and Integration* 4: 79–103.

Daenzer, Patricia M. 1992. "Ideology and the Formation of Migration Policy: The Case of Immigrant Domestic Workers, 1940–1990." Ph.D. diss., University of Toronto.

———. 1993. *Regulating Class Privilege: Immigrant Servants in Canada, 1940s–1990s.* Toronto: Scholars Press.

———. 1997. "An Affair between Nations: International Relations and the Movement of Household Service Workers." In *Not One of the Family: Foreign Domestic Workers in Canada*, edited by Abigail Bess Bakan and Daiva K. Stasiulis, 81–118. Toronto: University of Toronto Press.

Dancy, Joseph, and Penny A. Ralston. 2002. "Health Promotion and Black Elders: Subgroups of Greatest Need." *Research on Aging* 24(2): 218–242.

Das, Ajit, and Sharon Kemp. 1997. "Between Two Worlds: Counselling South Asian Americans." *Journal of Multicultural Counselling and Development* 25: 23–33.

Das, Veena. 2007. *Life and Words: Violence and the Descent into the Ordinary.* Berkeley: University of California Press.

Dei, George J. Sefa. 1992. "A Ghanaian Town Revisited: Changes and Continuities in Local Adaptive Strategies." *African Affairs* 91(362): 95–120.

Delgado, Richard. 1988. "Storytelling for Oppositionists and Others: A Plea for Narrative." *Michigan Law Review* 87: 2411–2441. Available at http://dx.doi.org/10.2307/1289308, accessed July 8, 2014.

———. 1995. "Words That Wound: A Tort Action for Racial Insults, Epithets, and Name Calling." In *Critical Race Theory: The Cutting Edge*, edited by Richard Delgado, 159–168. Philadelphia: Temple University Press.

Delgado, Richard, and Jean Stefancic, eds. 2012. *Critical Race Theory: An Introduction.* 2nd ed. New York: New York University Press.

Deneva, Neda. 2012. "Transnational Aging Carers: On Transformation of Kinship and Citizenship in the Context of Migration among Bulgarian Muslims to Spain." *Social Politics* 19(1): 105–128.

———. 2013. "Assembling Fragmented Citizenship: Bulgarian Muslim Migrants at the Margins of Two States." Ph.D. diss., Central European University.

———. 2015. "Conflicting Meanings and Practices of Work: Bulgarian Roma as Citizens and Migrants." In *Situating Migration in Transition: Temporal, Structural, and Conceptual*

Transformations of Migrations, edited by Raia Apostolova, Neda Deneva, and Tsvetelina Hristova, 42–70. Sofia: KOI.

Department of Immigration and Citizenship (DIAC). 2012–2013. "2012–13 Migration Program Report." Available at http://www.border.gov.au/ReportsandPublications/Documents/annual-reports/2012-13-diac-annual-report.pdf accessed October 27, 2015.

Diamond, Timothy. 1992. *Making Gray Gold: Narratives of Nursing Home Care.* Chicago: University of Chicago Press.

Di Leonardo, Micaela. 1987. "The Female World of Cards and Holidays: Women, Families, and the Work of Kinship." *Signs* 12(3): 440–453.

Doh, Daniel. 2012. *Exploring Social Protection Arrangements for Older People: Evidence from Ghana.* Saarbrücken, Germany: LAP Lambert Academic Press.

Dossa, Parin. 1999. "(Re)imagining Aging Lives: Ethnographic Narratives of Muslim Women in Diaspora." *Journal of Cross-Cultural Gerontology* 14(3): 245–272.

———. 2004. Politics and Poetics of Migration: Narratives of Iranian Women from The Diaspora. Canadian Scholar's Press, Ontario: Canada.

———. 2014. *Afghanistan Remembers: Gendered Narrations of Violence and Culinary Practices.* Toronto: University of Toronto Press.

Dreby, Joanna. 2010. *Divided by Borders: Mexican Migrants and Their Children.* Berkeley: University of California Press.

Dreby, Joanna, and Timothy Adkins. 2010. "Inequalities in Transnational Families." *Sociology Compass* 4: 673–689.

Dsane, Sarah. 2013. *Changing Cultures and Care of the Elderly.* Saarbrücken, Germany: LAP Lambert Academic Press.

Elder, Glen H., Jr. 1994. "Time, Human Agency, and Social Change: Perspectives on the Life Course." *Social Psychology Quarterly* 57: 4–15.

———. 1998. "Life Course and Human Development." In *Handbook of Child Psychology*, edited by W. Damon, 939–991. New York: Wiley.

Elder, Glen H., Jr., and Monica Johnson. 2002. "The Life Course and Aging: Challenges, Lessons, and New Directions." In *Invitation to the Life Course: Toward New Understanding of Later Life*, Pt. 2, edited by R. A. Settersten, Jr., 49–81. New York: Baywood Publishing.

Elliott, Louise. 2012. "Reunification 'Super Visas' Popular Despite Cost Concerns." *CBC News.* Available at http://www.cbc.ca/news/politics/reunification-super-visas-popular-despite-cost-concerns-1.1287439, accessed January 3, 2015.

Este, David C. 2004. "The Black Church as a Social Welfare Institution: Union United Church and the Development of Montreal's Black Community, 1907–1940." *Journal of Black Studies* 35(1): 3–22.

Estes, Caroll, Simon Biggs, and Chris Phillipson. 2010. *Social Theory, Social Policy, and Ageing: Critical Perspectives.* Maidenhead, UK: Open University Press.

European Commission. 1998. "Communication of the Commission on Undeclared Work." COM (98) 219, Brussels. Available at http://aei.pitt.edu/5111/1/5111.pdf, accessed October 17, 2015.

Evans, Bronwynne C., Neva Crogan, Michael Belyea, and David Coon. 2008. Utility of the Life Course Perspective in Research with Mexican American Caregivers of Older Adults. *Journal of Transcultural Nursing.* 20(1): 5–14.

Evans-Winters, Venus E., and Jennifer Esposito. 2010. "Other People's Daughters: Critical Race Feminism and Black Girls' Education." *Educational Foundations* 24: 11–24.

Fassin, Didier. 2007. *When Bodies Remember: Experiences and Politics of AIDS in South Africa.* Berkeley: University of California Press.

Fedyuk, Olena. 2011. "Beyond Motherhood: Ukrainian Female Labor Migration to Italy." Ph.D. diss., Central European University.

Fernández, Lillia. 2002. "Telling Stories about School: Using Critical Race Theory and Latino Critical Theories to Document Latina/Latino Education and Resistance." *Qualitative Inquiry* 8(1): 45–65.

Fesenmyer, Leslie. 2016. "'Assistance but Not Support': Pentecostalism and the Reconfiguring of Relatedness between Kenya and the United Kingdom." In *Affective Circuits: African Migrations to Europe and the Pursuit of Social Regeneration*, edited by Jennifer Cole and Christian Groes-Green, 125–145. Chicago: University of Chicago Press.

Few, April L. 2007. "Integrating Black Consciousness and Critical Race Feminism into Family Studies Research." *Journal of Family Issues* 28(4): 452–473.

Field, Dorothy, and Meredith Minkler. 1988. "Continuity and Change in Social Support between Young-Old and Old-Old or Very-Old Age." *Journal of Gerontology* 43(4):100–106.

Figueroa, Ester, and Patrick, Peter L. 2002. "The Meaning of Kiss-Teeth." Available at http://privatewww.essex.ac.uk/~patrickp/papers/KSTpapwww.pdf accessed June 7, 2015.

Finch, Janet, and Jennifer Mason. 1993. *Negotiating Family Commitments.* London: Tavistock/Routledge.

Fisher, Berenice, and Joan Tronto. 1990. "Toward a Feminist Theory of Caring." In *Circles of Care: Work and Identity in Women's Lives*, edited by Emily K. Abel and Margaret K. Nelson, 35–62. Albany: State University of New York Press.

Fitzpatrick, Meagan. 2013. "Don't Bring Parents Here for Welfare, Kenney Says: Immigration Minister Cites 'Abuse of Canada's Generosity' As Changes to Family Reunification Program Announced." *CBC News.* Available at http://www.cbc.ca/news/politics/don-t-bring-parents-here-for-welfare-kenney-says-1.1351002, accessed January 3, 2015.

Folbre, Nancy. 2001. *The Invisible Heart: Economics and Family Values.* New York: The New Press.

———. 2008. *Valuing Children: Rethinking the Economics of the Family.* Cambridge, MA: Harvard University Press.

Foner, Nancy. 2009. "Gender and Migration: West Indians in Comparative Perspective." *International Migration* 47(1): 3–29.

Foroohar, Rana. 2014. "2030: The Year Retirement Ends. Why We Need to Start Fixing It Now." *Time* 183(25): 40–44.

Fortes, Meyer. 1984. "Age, Generation, and Social Structure." In *Age and Anthropological Theory*, edited by David I. Kertzer and Jennie Keith, 99–122. Ithaca, NY: Cornell University Press.

Foucault, Michel. 1972. *The Archaeology of Knowledge.* New York: Pantheon.

Fouron, Georges E., and Nina Glick Schiller. 2002. "The Generation of Identity: Redefining the Second Generation within a Transnational Social Field." In *The Changing Face of Home: The Transnational Lives of the Second Generation*, edited by Georges E. Fouron and Mary C. Waters, 168–208. New York: Russell Sage Foundation.

Freidenberg, Judith Noemi. 2000. *Growing Old in El Barrio.* New York: New York University Press.

Friedman, Sara. 2006. *Intimate Politics.* Cambridge, MA: Harvard University Asia Center.

Funk, Laura, and Karen Kobayashi. 2009. "'Choice' in Filial Care Work: Moving beyond a Dichotomy." *Canadian Review of Sociology* 46(3): 236–252.

Gardner, Katy. 2002. *Age, Narrative, and Migration: The Life Course and Life Histories of Bengali Elders in London.* New York: Berg.

Gardner, Katy, and Ralph Grillo. 2002. "Transnational Households and Ritual: An Overview." *Global Networks* 2(3): 179–90.

Garro, Linda C., and Cheryl Mattingly. 2000. *Narrative and the Cultural Construction of Illness and Healing.* Berkeley: University of California Press.

Gee, Ellen, and Barbara Mitchell. 2003. "One Roof: Exploring Multi-generational Households in Canada." In *Voices: Essays on Canadian Families,* edited by M. Lynn, 293–313. 2nd ed. Toronto: Thomson Nelson.

George, Usha. 1998. "Caring and Women of Colour: Living the Intersecting Oppressions of Race, Class, and Gender." In *Women's Caring: Feminist Perspectives on Social Welfare,* edited by Carol Baines, Patricia Evans, and Sharon Neysmith, 69–93. Oxford: Oxford University Press.

Georges, Eugenia. 1990. *The Making of a Transnational Community: Migration, Development, and Cultural Change in the Dominican Republic.* New York: Columbia University Press.

Geronimus, Arlene T., Margaret Hicken, Danya Keene, and John Bound. 2006. "'Weathering' and Age Patterns of Allostatic Load Scores among Blacks and Whites in the United States." *American Journal of Public Health* 96(5): 826–833.

Gibson-Graham, J. K. 2006. *A Postcapitalist Politics.* Minneapolis: University of Minnesota Press.

Giesbrecht, Melissa. 2014. "Intersectionality and the 'Place' of Palliative Care Policy in British Columbia, Canada." Institute for Intersectionality Research and Policy. Simon Fraser University, Department of Geography. Available at http://www.sfu.ca/iirp/documents/ibpa/4_palliative_care_giesbrecht%202012.pdf, accessed October 31, 2015.

Gilbertson, Greta. 2009. "Caregiving across Generations: Aging, State Assistance, and Multigenerational Ties among Immigrants from the Dominican Republic." In *Across Generations: Immigrant Families in America,* edited by Nancy Foner, 135–160. New York: New York University Press.

Glenn, Evelyn Nakano. 1992. "From Servitude to Service Work: Historical Continuities in the Racial Division of Paid Reproductive Labor." *Signs* 18(1): 1–43.

———. 2010. *Forced to Care: Coercion and Caregiving in America.* Cambridge, MA: Harvard University Press.

Goody, Esther N. 1982. *Parenthood and Social Reproduction: Fostering and Occupational Roles in West Africa.* Cambridge: Cambridge University Press.

Gotanda, Neil. 1991. "A Critique of 'Our Constitution Is Colour-blind.'" *Stanford Law Review* 44: 1–68. Available at http://dx.doi.org/doi10.2307/1228940, accessed April 8, 2016.

Gottlieb, Alma. 2004. *The Afterlife Is Where We Come From: The Culture of Infancy in West Africa.* Chicago: University of Chicago Press.

Greenberg, Jessica, and Andrea Muhlebach. 2007. "The Old World and the New Economy: Notes on the 'Third Age' in Western Europe Today." In *Generations and Globalization,* edited by Jennifer Cole and Deborah Durham, 190–213. Bloomington: Indiana University Press.

Greenhalgh, Susan. 2010. "Governing Chinese Life: From Sovereignty to Biopolitical Governance." In *Governance of Life in Chinese Moral Experience: The Quest for an Adequate Life,* edited by Everett Yuehong Zhang, Arthur Kleinman, and Weiming Tu, 146–162. New York: Routledge.

Grewal, Sukhdev, Joan Bottorff, and Lynda Balneaves. 2004. "A Pap Test Screening Clinic in a South Asian Community of Vancouver, British Columbia: Challenges to Maintaining Utilization." *Public Health Nursing* 21(5): 412–418.

Grover, Shyam. 1978. "Temples." *India Abroad* October 8: 14.

Gubrium, Jaber F. 1975. *Living and Dying at Murray Manor.* New York: St. Martin's Press.

Gubrium, Jaber F., James A. Holstein, and David R. Buckholdt. 1994. *Constructing the Life Course.* Dix Hills, NY: General Hall.

Gulati, Leela, and Irudaya Rajan. 1999. "The Added Years: Elderly in India and Kerala." *Economic and Political Weekly* 34(44): WS-46–51.

Gunter, Lorne. 2011. "Immigrants Can't Expect to Bring Parents to Canada." *Calgary Herald*, October 24. Available at www.calgaryherald.com/opinion/Gunter+Immigrants+expect+bring+parents+Canada/5598728/story.html?cid=megadrop_story, accessed December 20, 2011.

Guo, Jinhua, and Arthur Kleinman. 2011. "Stigma HIV/AIDS, Mental Illness, and China's Nonpersons." In *Deep China*, edited by Arthur Kleinman et al., 237–262. Berkeley: University of California Press.

Gupta, Rashmi, and Vijayan Pillai. 2002. "Elder Caregiving in South Asian Families: Implications for Service." *Journal of Comparative Family Studies* 33(4): 565–576.

Hahamovitch, Cindy. 2011. *No Man's Land: Jamaican Guestworkers in America and the Global History of Deportable Labor*. Princeton, NJ: Princeton University Press.

Hamann, Edmund T., and Victor Zúñiga. 2011. "Schooling and the Everyday Ruptures Transnational Children Encounter in the United States and Mexico." In *Everyday Ruptures: Children, Youth, and Migration in Global Perspective*, edited by Cati Coe, Rachel R. Reynolds, Deborah A. Boehm, Julia Meredith Hess, and Heather Rae-Espinoza, 141–161. Nashville, TN: Vanderbilt University Press.

Han, J. P. 2005. "Please Value Our Parents: Exploration of the Problems Related to Elderly (Chinese) Immigrants." In Chinese. *Singdao Daily*, A7.

Hancock, Linda. 1999. "Citizenship on the Margins: The Case of Divorce in Western Europe." In *Citizenship and Identity in Europe*, edited by Leslie Holmes and Philomena Murray, 97–119. Aldershot: Ashgate.

Hareven, Tamara K. 1994. "Aging and Generational Relations: A Historical and Life Course Perspective." *Annual Review of Sociology* 20: 437–461.

Hazan, Haim. 1992. *Managing Change in Old Age: The Control of Meaning in an Institutional Setting*. Albany: State University of New York Press.

Hennock, E. P. 2007. *The Origin of the Welfare State in England and Germany, 1850–1914*. Cambridge: Cambridge University Press.

Henry, Frances. 1994. *The Caribbean Diaspora in Toronto: Learning to Live with Racism*. Toronto: University of Toronto Press.

Heyse, Paul. 2011. "A Life Course Perspective in the Analysis of Self-Experiences of Female Migrants in Belgium: The Case of Ukrainian and Russian Women in Belgium." *Migration* 27(2): 199–225.

Hill, Polly. 1963. *The Migrant Cocoa-Farmers of Southern Ghana: A Study in Rural Capitalism*. Cambridge: Cambridge University Press.

———. 2003. *The Commercialization of Intimate Life: Notes from Home and Work*. Berkeley: University of California Press.

Holmes, Douglas R. 1989. *Cultural Disenchantments: Worker Peasantries in Northeast Italy*. Princeton, NJ: Princeton University Press.

Hondagneu-Sotelo, Pierrette. 2007. *Doméstica: Immigrant Workers Cleaning and Caring in the Shadows of Affluence*. Berkeley: University of California Press.

Hondagneu-Sotelo, Pierrette, and Ernestine Avila. 1997. "'I'm Here, but I'm There': The Meanings of Latina Transnational Motherhood." *Gender and Society* 11(5): 548–571.

Horton, Sarah. 2009. "A Mother's Heart Is Weighted Down with Stones: A Phenomenological Approach to the Experience of Transnational Motherhood." *Culture, Medicine, and Psychiatry* 33: 21–40.

Houh, Emily M. S., and Kristin Kalsem. 2015. "Theorizing Legal Participatory Action Research Critical Race/Feminism and Participatory Action Research." *Qualitative Inquiry* 21(3): 262–276.

Houle, Leta. 2011. "Issues of Tension: Aboriginal Women and Western Feminism." *Religious Studies and Theology* 30(2): 209–233.

Hu, Bi Ying, and Judit Szente. 2009. "The Care and Education of Orphan Children with Disabilities in China: Progress and Remaining Challenges." *Childhood Education* 86(2): 78–86.

Hutchison, Elizabeth D. 2010. *Dimensions of Human Behavior: The Changing Life Course.* Thousand Oaks, CA: Sage Publications.

Hwang, Eunju. 2008. "Exploring Aging-in-Place among Chinese and Korean Seniors in British Columbia, Canada." *Ageing International* 32: 205–218.

Igarashi, Heidi, Karen Hooker, Deborah Coehlo, and Margaret Manoogian. 2013. "'My Nest Is Full': Intergenerational Relationships at Midlife." *Journal of Aging Studies* 27(2): 102–112.

Ikels, Charlotte, ed. 2004. *Filial Piety.* Stanford, CA: Stanford University Press.

ILO. 2002. *Decent Work and the Informal Economy.* Geneva: International Labour Office.

Isastia, Anna Maria 1991. "L'emigrazione italiana in Australia." In *Italia-Australa, 1788–1988,* edited by R. Ugolini, 203–252. Rome: Edizioni del l'Ateneo.

Iuliano, Susanna. 2010. *Vite Italiane: Italian Lives in Western Australia.* Nedlands, Australia: University of Western Australia Publishing.

Jacka, Tamara. 2009. "Cultivating Citizens: Suzhi Discourse (Quality) in the PRC." *Positions: East Asia Culture Critique* 17(3): 523–535.

James, Carl E. 2009. "African-Caribbean Canadians Working 'Harder' to Attain Their Immigrant Dreams: Context, Strategies, and Consequences." *Wadabagei: A Journal of the Caribbean and Its Diaspora* 12(1): 92–108.

James, Carl E., David Este, Wanda Thomas Bernard, Akua Benjamin, Bethan Lloyd, and Tana Turner. 2010. *Race and Well-being: The Lives, Hopes, and Activism of African Canadians.* Halifax, Canada: Fernwood Publishing.

Jasso, Guillermina. 2003. "Migration, Human Development, and the Life Course." In *Handbook of the Life Course.* edited by Jeyaln T. Mortimer and Michael J. Shanahan, 331–364. New York: Kluwer Academic/Plenum Publishers.

Jileva, Elena. 2002. "Visa and Free Movement of Labour: The Uneven Imposition of the EU Acquis on the Accession States." *Journal of Ethnic and Migration Studies* 28(4):683–700.

Kang, Jennifer Yusun. 2012. "How Do Narrative and Language Skills Relate to Each Other? Investigation of Young Korean EFL Learners' Oral Narratives." *Narrative Inquiry* 22(2): 307–331.

Karatzogianni, Athina, and Adi Kuntsman, eds. 2012. *Digital Cultures and the Politics of Emotion: Feelings, Affect, and Technological Change.* Basingstoke, UK: Palgrave.

Kauh, Tae-Ock. 1997. "Intergenerational Relations: Older Korean-Americans' Experiences." *Journal of Cross-Cultural Gerontology* 12: 245–271.

———. 1998. "Changing Status and Roles of Older Korean Immigrants in the United States." *International Journal of Aging and Human Development* 49: 213–229.

Keefe, Janice, and Pamela Fancey. 2002. "Work and Eldercare: Reciprocity between Older Mothers and Their Employed Daughters." *Canadian Journal on Aging* 21(2): 229–241.

Keith, Jennie, and David I. Kertzer. 1984. "Introduction." In *Age and Anthropological Theory,* edited by Kertzer and Keith, 19–61. Ithaca, NY: Cornell University Press.

Kennedy, Paul, and Victor Roudometof, eds. 2002. *Communities across Borders: New Immigrants and Transnational Cultures.* New York: Routledge.

Keyser, Catherine. 2009. "The Role of the State and NGOs in Caring for At-Risk Children: The Case of Orphan Care." In *State and Society Responses to Welfare Needs in China: Serving the People,* edited by Jonathan Schwartz and Shawn Hsieh, 45–65. New York: Routledge.

Khatusky, Galina, Joshua M. Weiner, and Wayne L. Anderson. 2010. "Immigrant and Non-Immigrant Certified Nursing Assistants in Nursing Homes: How Do They Differ?" *Journal of Aging and Social Policy* 22(3): 267–287.

Kilkey, Majella, and Laura Merla. 2014. "Situating Transnational Families' Care giving Arrangements: The Role of Institutional Contexts." *Global Networks* 14(2): 210–229.

Kleinman, Arthur, Yunxiang Yan, Jing Jun, Sing Lee, Everett Zhang, Pan Tianshu, Wu Fei, and Guo Jinhua, eds. 2011. *Deep China*. Berkeley: University of California Press.

Klocke-Daffa, Sabine. 2014. "Contested Claims to Social Welfare: Basic Income Grants in Namibia." Paper presented at workshop on Social Policy and Regimes of Social Welfare in Africa, University of Fribourg, Fribourg, Switzerland, September.

Koehn, Sharon. 2009. "Negotiating Candidacy: Access to Care for Ethnic Minority Seniors." *Ageing and Society* 29(4): 585–608.

Kofman, Eleonore. 2012. "Rethinking Care through Social Reproduction: Articulating Circuits of Migration." *Social Politics* 19(1): 142–162.

Kraler, Albert, Eleonore Kofman, Martin Kohli, and Camille Schmoll, eds. 2011. *Gender, Generations, and the Family in International Migration*. Amsterdam: Amsterdam University Press.

Kwan, Mei-Po. 2007. "Affecting Geospatial Technologies." *The Professional Geographer* 59(1): 22–34.

Ladson-Billings, Gloria, and William F. Tate IV. 1995. "Toward a Critical Race Theory of Education." *Teachers College Record* 97(1): 47–68.

Lai, Daniel W. L. 2004. "Depression among Elderly Chinese-Canadian Immigrants from Mainland China." *Chinese Medical Journal* 117: 677–683.

Lai, Daniel W. L., and Wendy L. Leonenko. 2007. "Correlates of Living Alone among Single Elderly Chinese Immigrants in Canada." *International Journal of Aging and Human Development* 65: 121–148.

Lamb, Sarah. 2002. "Intimacy in a Transnational Era: The Remaking of Aging among Indian Americans." *Diaspora: A Journal of Transnational Studies* 11(3): 299–330.

———. 2007. "Aging across Worlds: Modern Seniors in an Indian Diaspora." In *Generations and Globalization: Youth, Age, and Family in the New World Economy*, edited by Jennifer Cole and Deborah Lynn Durham, 132–163. Bloomington: Indiana University Press.

———. 2009. *Aging and the Indian Diaspora: Cosmopolitan Families in India and Abroad*. Bloomington: Indiana University Press.

———. 2014. "Permanent Personhood or Meaningful Decline? Toward a Critical Anthropology of Successful Aging." *Journal of Aging Studies* 29: 41–52.

Lamphere, Louise, Alex Stepick, and Guillermo Grenier, eds. 1994. *Newcomers in the Workplace: Immigrants and the Restructuring of the U.S. Economy*. Philadelphia: Temple University Press.

Lan, Pei-Cha. 2002. "Subcontracting Filial Piety: Elder Care in Ethnic Chinese Immigrant Families in California." *Journal of Family Issues* 23: 812–835.

Lancaster, Roger N. 1992. *Life Is Hard: Machismo, Danger, and the Intimacy of Power in Nicaragua*. Berkeley: University of California Press.

Lang, Fu. 2006. "Yimin Haiwai hou, fumu zinv jian de qingqin zengmo bianle weier [Why has the relationship between parents and children changed after immigration]." Available at http://www.wenxuecity.com/news/2006/07/27/-285864.html, accessed May 23, 2007.

Laungani, Pittu. 2005. "Changing Patterns of Family Life in India." In *Families in Global Perspective*, edited by J. P. Roopnarine and U. P. Gielen, 85–103. Boston: Pearson Education.

Lawson, Erica. 2013. "The Gendered Working Lives of Seven Jamaican Women in Canada: A Story about 'Here' and 'There' in a Transnational Economy." *Feminist Formations* 25(1): 138–156.

Laz, Cheryl. 1998. "Act Your Age." *Sociological Forum* 13(1): 85–113.

Leach, Belinda. 2013. "Canada's Migrants without History: Neoliberal Immigration Regimes and Trinidadian Transnationalism." *International Migration* 51(2): 32–45.

Leung, Ho Hon, and Lynn McDonald. 2007. "Chinese Women Who Care for Ageing Parents in Three-Generational Households: Some Immigrant Experiences in Toronto." *Asian Journal of Gerontology and Geriatrics* 2(1): 15–22.

Leutz, Walter N. 2007. "Immigration and the Elderly: Foreign-Born Workers in Long-Term Care." *Immigration Policy in Focus* 5(12): 1–11.

Levitt, Peggy. 1998. "Social Remittances: Migration-Driven Local-Level Forms of Cultural Diffusion." *International Migration Review* 32(4): 926–948.

Levitt, Peggy, and Nina Glick Schiller. 2004. "Conceptualizing Simultaneity: A Transnational Social Field Perspective on Society." *International Migration Review* 38(3): 1002–1039.

Li, Hongshi. 2009. "'Little Quilted Vests to Warm Parents' Hearts': Redefining the Gendered Practice of Filial Piety in Rural North-eastern China." *The China Quarterly* 198: 348–363.

Li, Peter S. 2011. "Immigrants from China to Canada: Issues of Supply and Demand of Human Capital." In *Migration, Indigenization, and Interaction: Chinese Overseas and Globalization*, edited by L. Suryadinata, 73–95. Hackensack, NJ: World Scientific Publishing.

Lie, Mabel L. S. 2010. "Across the Oceans: Childcare and Grandparenting in UK Chinese and Bangladeshi Households." *Journal of Ethnic and Migration Studies* 36: 1425–1443.

Lincoln, Yvonna, and Egon Guba. 1985. *Naturalistic Inquiry.* Newbury Park, CA: Sage Publications.

Liu, Haiming. 2006. *Transnational History of a Chinese Family: Immigrant Letters, Family Business, and Reverse Migration.* New Brunswick, NJ: Rutgers University Press.

Livingston, Julie. 2005. *Debility and the Moral Imagination in Botswana.* Bloomington: Indiana University Press.

Lloyd-Sherlock, Peter, Armando Barrientos, Valerie Moller, and João Saboia. 2012. "Pensions, Poverty, and Well-Being in Later Life: Comparative Research from Brazil and South Africa." *Journal of Aging Studies* 26(3): 243–252.

Lock, Margaret. 1995. *Encounters with Aging: Medicalization of Menopause in Japan and North America.* Berkeley: University of California Press.

Lomnitz, Larissa Adler. 1977. *Networks and Marginality: Life in a Mexican Shantytown.* New York: Academic Press.

Love, Barbara, J. 2004. "Brown Plus Counter-Storytelling: A Critical Race Theory Analysis of the Majoritarian Achievement Gap Story." *Equity and Excellence in Education* 37: 227–246.

Lunt, Neil. 2009. "Older People within Transnational Families: The Social Policy Implications." *International Journal of Social Welfare* 18: 243–251.

Lutz, Helma, ed. 2007. *Migration and Domestic Work: A European Perspective on a Global Theme.* Studies in Migration and Diaspora. Aldershot, UK: Ashgate.

———. 2010. "Gender in the Migratory Process." *Journal of Ethnic and Migration Studies* 36(10): 1647–1663.

MacKinnon, Catherine A. 1983. "Feminism, Marxism, Method, and the State: Toward Feminist Jurisprudence." *Signs* 8(4): 635–658.

———. 1993. "Reflections on Law in the Everyday Life of Women." In *Law in Everyday Life*, edited by Austin Sarat and Thomas R. Kearns, 109–122. Ann Arbor: University of Michigan Press.

Madianou, Mirca. 2016. "Ambient Co-presence: Transnational Family Practices in Polymedia Environments." *Journal of Global Networks* 16: 183–201.

Madianou, Mirca, and Daniel Miller. 2012. *Migration and the New Media: Transnational Families and Polymedia.* New York: Routledge.

Maher, Jane M., Jo Lindsay, and Suzanne Franzway. 2008. "Time, Caring Labour, and Social Policy: Understanding the Family Time Economy in Contemporary Families." *Work, Employment, and Society* 22(3): 547–558.

Mahler, Sarah J. 1995. *American Dreaming: Immigrant Life on the Margins.* Princeton, NJ: Princeton University Press.

Mahmood, Saba. 2011. *Politics of Piety: The Islamic Revival and the Feminist Subject.* Princeton, NJ: Princeton University Press.

Mamdani, Mahmood. 1996. *Citizen and Subject: Contemporary Africa and the Legacy of Late Colonialism.* Princeton, NJ: Princeton University Press.

Man, Guida. 2002. "Globalization and the Erosion of the Welfare State: Effects on Chinese Women." *Canadian Women Studies* 21/22(4/1): 26–32.

Mancheva, Mila, and Evgenia Troeva. 2011. "Migrations to and from Bulgaria: The State of Research." In *Migrations, Gender and Intercultural Integration in Bulgaria*, edited by Georgeta Nazarska and Marko Hajdinjak, 13–60. Sofia, Bulgaria: IMIR.

Mannheim, Karl. [1952] 1972. "The Problem of Generations." In *Essays on the Sociology of Knowledge*, 276–322. London: Routledge and Kegan Paul.

Manuh, Takyiwaa. 2006. *An 11th Region of Ghana? Ghanaians Abroad.* Accra, Ghana: Ghana Academy of Arts and Sciences.

Mareschal, Patrice. 2006. "Innovation and Adaptation: Contrasting Efforts to Organize Home Care Workers in Four States." *Labor Studies Journal* 31(1): 25–49.

———. 2007. "How the West Was Won: An Inside View of the SEIU's Strategies and Tactics for Organizing Home Care Workers in Oregon." *International Journal of Organization Theory and Behavior* 10(3): 387–412.

Markova, Eugenia. 2010. "Legal Status and Migrant Economic Performance: The Case of Bulgarians in Spain and Greece." In *Bulgaria and Europe: Shifting Identities*, edited by Stefanos Katsikasm, 91–112. London and New York: Anthem.

Mason, Jennifer. 2004. "Managing Kinship over Long Distances: The Significance of the 'Visit.'" *Social Policy and Society* 3: 421–429.

Massey-Dozier, Jody. 2011. "I Earns My Struttin' Shoes: Blues Women and Leadership." In *Black Womanist Leadership: Tracing the Motherline*, edited by Toni C. King and Alease A Fugerson, 113–122. Albany: State University of New York Press.

Masvie, Hilde. 2006. "The Role of Tamang Mothers-in-Law in Promoting Breast Feeding in Makwanpur District, Nepal." *Midwifery* 22(1): 23–31.

Matsuda, Mari J. 1991. "Voices of America: Accent, Antidiscrimination Law, and a Jurisprudence for the Last Reconstruction." *Yale Law Journal* 100(5): 1329–1407.

Mattingly, Cheryl. 2014. *Moral Laboratories: Family Peril and the Struggle for a Good Life.* Berkeley: University of California Press.

Mauss, Marcel. 1990. *The Gift: The Form and Reason for Exchange in Archaic Societies*, translated by W. G. Halls. New York: Routledge.

Mazzucato, Valentina. 2008a. "Transnational Reciprocity: Ghanaian Migrants and the Care of Their Parents Back Home." In *Generations in Africa: Connections and Conflicts*, edited by Erdmute Alber, Sjaak van der Geest, and Susan R. Whyte, III–133. Münster, Germany: Lit Verlag.

———. 2008b. "Informal Insurance Arrangements in Ghanaian Migrants' Transnational Networks: The Role of Reverse Remittances and Geographic Proximity." *World Development* 37(6): 1105–1115.

Mazzucato, Valentina, and Djamila Schans. 2011. "Transnational Families and the Well-being of Children: Conceptual and Methodological Challenges." *Journal of Marriage and Family* 73: 704–712.

McGlynn, Clare. 2000. "A Family Law for the European Union." In *Social Law and Policy in an Evolving European Union*, edited by Jo Shaw, 233–242. Oxford: Hart Publishing.

———. 2001. "Families and the European Charter of Fundamental Rights: Progressive Change or Entrenching the Status Quo?" *European Law Review* 26(6): 582–598.

Meillassoux, Claude. 1972. "From Reproduction to Production." *Economy and Society* 1: 95–105.

———. 1981. *Maidens, Meal, and Money: Capitalism and the Domestic Community*. Cambridge: Cambridge University Press.

Merrifield, A. 2006. *Henri Lefebvre: A Critical Introduction*. London: Routledge.

Michel, Sonya, and Rianne Mahon, eds. 2002. *Child Care Policy at the Crossroads: Gender and Welfare State Restructuring*. New York: Psychology Press.

Miller, Daniel. 2008. *The Comfort of Things*. Cambridge: Polity Press.

Mitchell, Barbara A. 2007. *The Boomerang Age: Transitions to Adulthood in Families*. New Brunswick, NJ: Transaction Publishers.

Monture, Patrica. 2010. "Race, Gender, and the University: Strategies for Survival." In *States of Race: Critical Race Feminism for the 21st Century*, edited by Sherene Razack, Sunera Thobani, and Malinda Smith, 23–36. Toronto: Between the Lines.

Moore, Henrietta L. 1988. *Feminism and Anthropology*. Minneapolis: University of Minnesota Press.

Morokvasic, Mirjana. 1983. "Women in Migration: Beyond the Reductionist Outlook." In *One Way Ticket: Migration and Female Labour*, edited by Annie Phizacklea, 13–31. London: Routledge and Kegan Paul.

———. 2004. "'Settled in Mobility': Engendering Post-Wall Migration in Europe." *Feminist Review* 77(1): 7–25.

Mullings, Delores V. 2004. "Situating Older Caribbean Canadian Women in Feminist Research: A Reflection." *Canadian Woman Studies* 23(2): 134–139.

———. 2010. "Temporary Mothering: Grieving the Loss of Foster Children When They Leave." *Journal of the Motherhood Initiative for Research and Community Involvement* 1(2): 165–176.

———. 2013. "How Black Mothers 'Successfully' Raise Children in the 'Hostile' Canadian Climate." *Journal of the Motherhood Initiative for Research and Community Involvement* 4(2): 105–119.

———. 2015. "The Racial Institutionalization of Whiteness in Contemporary Canadian Public Policy." In *Unveiling Whiteness in the 21st Century: Global Manifestations*, edited by Veronica Watson, Deirdre Howard-Wagner, and Lisa Spanierman, 115–140. New York: Lexington Books.

Murphy, Rachel. 2004. "Turning Peasants into Modern Chinese Citizens: 'Population Quality' Discourse, Demographic Transition, and Primary Education." *China Quarterly* 177: 1–20.

Murray, Colin. 1981. *Families Divided: The Impact of Migrant Labor in Lesotho*. Cambridge: Cambridge University Press.

Myerhoff, Barbara. 1978. *Number Our Days*. New York: E. F. Dutton.

Myerhoff, Barbara, and Lynne Littman. 1977. *Number Our Days*. DVD. Santa Monica: Direct Cinema Ltd.

Nazareno, Jennifer Pabelonia, Rhacel Salazar Parreñas, and Yu-Kang Fan. 2014. "Can I Ever Retire? The Plight of Migrant Filipino Elderly Caregivers in Los Angeles." Available at http://www.irle.ucla.edu/publications/documents/CanIEverRetirePolicyReportIRLE .pdf, accessed December 17, 2014.

Neugarten, Bernice L. 1974. "Age Groups in American Society and the Rise of the Young-Old." *Annals of the American Academy of Political and Social Science* 415(1): 187–198.

———. 1996. *The Meanings of Age: Selected Papers*. Chicago: University of Chicago Press.

Neumark, David, and Patrick Button. 2014. "Age Discrimination and the Great Recession." *FRBSF Economic Letter* 10: 1–5.

Ng, Cheuk Fan, Herbert Northcott, and Sharon Abu-Laban. 2007. "Housing and Living Arrangements of South Asian Immigrant Seniors in Edmonton, Alberta." *Canadian Journal on Aging* 26(3): 189–194.

Nichter, Mark. 2010. "Idioms of Distress Revisited." *Culture, Medicine, and Psychiatry* 34: 401–416.

Nyland, Berenice, Xiaodong Zeng, Chris Nyland, and Ly Tran. 2009. "Grandparents as Educators and Carers in China." *Journal of Early Childhood Research* 7(1): 46–57.

Olwig, Karen Fog. 1999. "Narratives of the Children Left Behind: Home and Identity in Globalised Caribbean Families." *Journal of Ethnic and Migration Studies* 25(2): 267–284.

———. 2002. "A Wedding in the Family: Home Making in a Global Kin Network." *Global Networks* 2(3): 205–218.

———. 2007. *Caribbean Journeys: An Ethnography of Migration and Home in Three Family Networks*. Durham, NC: Duke University Press.

———. 2012. "The Care Chain, Children's Mobility, and the Caribbean Migration Tradition." *Journal of Ethnic and Migration Studies* 38(6): 933–952.

Ong, Aihwa. 1995. "Making the Biopolitical Subject: Cambodian Immigrants, Refugee Medicine, and Cultural Citizenship in California." *Social Science and Medicine* 40(9): 1243–1257.

———. 1999. *Flexible Citizenship: The Cultural Logics of Transnationality*. Durham, NC: Duke University Press.

Ornstein, Michael D. 2000. *Ethno-racial Inequality in the City of Toronto: Analysis of the 1996 Census*. Toronto: Institute of Social Research, York University.

Ornstein, Michael D., and Raghubar D. Sharma. 1983. *Adjustment and Economic Experience of Immigrants in Canada: An Analysis of the 1976 Longitudinal Survey of Immigrants: A Report to Employment and Immigration Canada, April 1981*. Toronto: Institute for Behavioural Research, York University.

Ortner, Sherry B. 2006. *Anthropology and Social Theory: Culture, Power, and the Acting Subject*. Durham, NC: Duke University Press.

Paraprofessional Health Institute. 2014. "An Aging Direct-Care Workforce." Available at http://phinational.org/aging-direct-care-workforce, accessed December 16, 2014.

Parreñas, Rhacel Salazar. 2001. *Servants of Globalization: Women, Migration, and Domestic Work*. Stanford, CA: Stanford University Press.

———. 2004. *Children of Global Migration: Transnational Families and Gendered Woes*. Stanford, CA: Stanford University Press.

———. 2005. "Long Distance Intimacy: Class, Gender, and Intergenerational Relations between Mothers and Children in Filipino Transnational Families." *Global Networks* 5(4): 317–336.

Peterson, V. Spike. 2010. "Global Householding amid Global Crises." *Politics and Gender* 6(2): 271–281.

Plaza, Dwaine. 2004. "Disaggregating the Indo and African-Caribbean Migration and Settlement Experience in Canada." *Canadian Journal of Latin American and Caribbean Studies* 29(57–58): 241–266.

Portes, Alejandro. 2003. "Theoretical Convergences and Empirical Evidence in the Study of Immigrant Transnationalism." *International Migration Review* 37(3): 814–892.

Potter, Jack, and Sulamith Heins Potter. 1990. *China's Peasants: The Anthropology of a Revolution.* Cambridge: Cambridge University Press.

Poverty Fact Sheet. 2007. "Understanding the Racialization of Poverty in Ontario: An Introduction in 2007." Available at http://www.learningandviolence.net/lrnteach/material/PovertyFactSheets-aug07.pdf, accessed July 2, 2015.

Pupo, Norene, and Ann Duffy. 2003. "Caught in the Net: The Impact of Changes to Canadian Employment Insurance Legislation on Part-Time Workers." *Social Policy and Society* 2(1): 1–11.

Pyle, Jean. 2006. "Globalization and the Increase in Transnational Care Work: The Flip Side." *Globalizations* 3(3): 297–315.

Qi, Xiaoying. 2014. "Filial Obligation in Contemporary China: Evolution of the Culture-System." *Journal for the Theory of Social Behavior* 45(1): 141–161.

Rae-Espinoza, Heather. 2011. "The Children of Émigrés in Ecuador: Narratives of Cultural Reproduction and Emotion in Transnational Social Fields." In *Everyday Ruptures: Children, Youth, and Migration in Global Perspective*, edited by Cati Coe, Rachel R. Reynolds, Deborah A. Boehm, Julia Meredith Hess, and Heather Rae-Espinoza, 115–138. Nashville, TN: Vanderbilt University Press.

Razack, Sherene. 1998. *Looking White People in the Eye: Gender, Race, and Culture in Courtrooms and Classrooms.* Toronto: University of Toronto Press.

Redfoot, Donald L., and Ari N. Houser. 2005. "'We Shall Travel On': Quality of Care, Economic Development, and the International Migration of Long-Term Care Workers." Washington, DC: AARP Public Policy Institute.

Regis, Helen A. 2003. *Fulbe Voices: Marriage, Islam, and Medicine in Northern Cameroon.* Boulder, CO: Westview Press.

Richmond, Anthony H. 1993. "Education and Qualifications of Caribbean Migrants in Metropolitan Toronto." *Journal of Ethnic and Migration Studies* 19(2): 263–280.

Richmond, Anthony H., and Bali Ram. 1989. "Caribbean Immigrants: A Demo-Economic Analysis." Vol. 91. Ottawa: Statistics Canada.

Ries, Nancy. 2009. "Potato Ontology: Surviving Postsocialism in Russia." *Cultural Anthropology* 24(2): 181–212.

Ritchie, Jane, and Jane Lewis. 2003. *Qualitative Research Practice.* Thousand Oaks, CA: Sage Publishers.

Rocha, José Luis. 2006. *Una región desgarrada: Dinámicas migratorias en centroamérica.* San José, Costa Rica: Servicio Jesuita para Migrantes Centroamérica.

Rouse, Roger. 1992. "Making Sense of Settlement: Class Transformation, Cultural Struggle, and Transnationalism among Mexican Migrants in the United States." In *Towards a Transnational Perspective on Migration: Race, Class, Ethnicity, and Nationalism*, edited by Nina Glick Schiller, Linda Basch, and Cristina Blanc-Szanton, 25–52. New York: New York Academy of Sciences.

Rushdie, Salman. 1991. *Imaginary Homelands.* London: Granta Books.

Safa, Helen Icken. 1995. *The Myth of the Male Breadwinner: Women and Industrialization in the Caribbean.* Boulder. CO: Westview Press.

Safri, Maliha, and Julie Graham. 2010. "The Global Household: Toward a Feminist Postcapitalist International Political Economy." *Signs* 36(1): 99–125.

Sahlins, Marshall. 2004. *Apologies to Thucydides: Understanding History as Culture and Vice Versa*. Chicago: University of Chicago Press.

———. 2010. "What Kinship Is (Part One)." *Journal of the Royal Anthropological Institute* 17: 2–19.

———. 2011. "What Kinship Is (Part Two)." *Journal of the Royal Anthropological Institute* 17: 227–242.

Sassen, Saskia. 2000. "Women's Burden: Counter-Geographies of Globalization." *Journal of International Affairs* 53(2): 503–524.

———. 2014. *Expulsions: Brutality and Complexity in the Global Economy*. Cambridge, MA: Harvard University Press.

Schapera, Isaac. 1947. *Migrant Labour and Tribal Life: A Study of Conditions in the Bechuanaland Protectorate*. Oxford: Oxford University Press.

Schmalzbauer, Leah. 2004. "Searching for Wages and Mothering from Afar: The Case of Honduran Transnational Families." *Journal of Marriage and Family* 66: 1317–1331.

Scott, Katherine, Kevin Selbee, and Paul Reed. 2005. *Making Connections: Social and Civic Engagement among Canadian Immigrants*. Ottawa: Canadian Council for Social Development.

Sekyi, Kobina. 1974. *The Blinkards*. London: Heinemann Educational.

Settles, Barbara H., Jia Zhao, Karen Doneker Mancini, Amanda Rich, Shawnella Pierre, and Atieno Oduor. 2009. "Grandparents Caring for Grandchildren: Emerging Roles and Exchanges in Global Perspectives." *Journal of Comparative Family Studies* 40(5): 827–848.

Shang, Xiaoyuan. 2008. "The Role of Extended Families in Childcare and Protection: The Case of Rural China." *International Journal of Social Welfare* 17: 204–215.

———. 2010. *Zhongguo er tong fu li qian yan wen ti* [Discovery report: emerging issues and findings for child welfare and protection in China]. Beijing: China Social Sciences Academic Press.

Shang, Xiaoyuan, and Karen R. Fisher. 2013. *Caring for Orphaned Children in China*. Lexington Books.

Shang, Xiaoyuan, and Xiaoming Wu. 2011. "The Care Regime in China: Elder and Child Care." *Journal of Comparative Social Welfare* 27(2): 123–131.

Sharma, Rashmi, and Candace Kemp. 2012. "'One Should Follow the Wind': Individualized Filial Piety and Support Exchanges in Indian Immigrant Families in the United States." *Journal of Aging Studies* 26(2): 129–139.

Shipton, Parker. 2007. *The Nature of Entrustment: Intimacy, Exchange, and the Sacred in Africa*. New Haven: Yale University Press.

Sigley, Gary. 2009. "*Suzhi*, the Body, and the Fortunes of Technoscientific Reasoning in Contemporary China." *Positions: East Asia Cultures Critique* 17(3): 537–566.

Silvera, Makeda. 1989. *Silenced*. 2nd ed. Toronto: Sister Vision Press.

———. 1992. "Man Royals and Sodomites: Some Thoughts on the Invisibility of Afro-Caribbean Lesbians." *Feminist Studies* 18(3): 521–532.

Simic, Andrei. 1978. "Introduction: Aging and the Aged in Cultural Perspective." In *Life's Career—Aging: Cultural Variations on Growing Old*, edited by Barbara Myerhoff and Andrei Simic, 9–22. London: Sage Publications.

Simic, Andrei, and Barbara Myerhoff. 1978. "Conclusion." In *Life's Career—Aging: Cultural Variations on Growing Old*, edited by Myerhoff and Simic, 231–247. London: Sage Publications.

Simmons, Alan, and Dwaine Plaza. 2006. "The Caribbean Community in Canada: Transnational Connections and Transformations." In *Negotiating Borders and Belonging: Transnational Identities and Practices in Canada*, edited by Vic Satzewich and Lloyd Wong, 130–149. Vancouver: University of British Columbia Press.

Singh, Supriya, Anuja Cabraal, and Shanthi Robertson. 2010. "Remittances as a Currency of Care: A Focus on 'Twice Migrants' among the Indian Diaspora in Australia." *Journal of Comparative Family Studies* 41(2): 245–263.

Small, Cathy. 1997. *Voyages: From Tongan Villages to American Suburbs.* Ithaca, NY: Cornell University Press.

Smith, Kristin, and Reagan Baughman. 2007. "Caring for America's Aging Population: A Profile of the Direct-Care Workforce." *Monthly Labor Review* September: 20–26.

Solórzano, Daniel G., and Dolores Delgado Bernal. 2001. "Examining Transformational Resistance through a Critical Race and Latino Critical Theory Framework: Chicana and Chicano Students in an Urban Context." *Urban Education* 36(3): 308–342.

Solórzano, Daniel G., and Tara J. Yosso. 2001. Critical race and LatCrit theory and method: Counter-storytelling. *International Journal of Qualitative Studies in Education,* 14(4): 471–495.

———. 2002. "Critical Race Methodology: Counter-storytelling as an Analytical Framework for Education Research." *Qualitative Inquiry* 8(1): 23–44.

Somjee, Geeta. 1989. *Narrowing the Gender Gap.* London: Macmillan Press.

Spitzer, Denise, Anne Neufeld, Margaret Harrison, Karen Hughes, and Miriam Stewart. 2003. "Caregiving in Transnational Context: 'My Wings Have Been Cut; Where Can I Fly?'" *Gender and Society* 17(2): 267–286.

Stack, Carol. 1974. *All Our Kin: Strategies for Survival in a Black Community.* New York: Harper & Row.

———. 1996. *Call to Home: African Americans Reclaim the Rural South.* New York: Basic Books.

Stack, Carol, and Linda M. Burton. 1993. "Kinscripts." *Journal of Comparative Family Studies* 24(2): 157–170.

Stanley, Liz. 2010. "To the Letter: Thomas and Znaniecki's The Polish Peasant and Writing a Life, Sociologically." *Life Writing* 7(2): 139–151.

Statistics Canada. 2008. General Social Survey Cycle 21: Family. Ottawa, Ontario: 2007. Social Support and Retirement.

———. 2011. "Do Highly Educated Immigrants Perform Differently in the Canadian and U.S. Labour Markets?" Available at http://www.statcan.gc.ca/pub/11f0019m/2011329/part -partie1-eng.htm accessed May 14, 2014.

———. 2013. "Immigration and Ethnocultural Diversity in Canada." Available at http://www12.statcan.gc.ca/nhs-enm/2011/as-sa/99-010-x/99-010-x2011001-eng.cfm accessed April 12, 2014.

Stephen, Lynn. 2007. *Transborder Lives: Indigenous Oaxacans in Mexico, California, and Oregon.* Durham, NC: Duke University Press.

Stepick, Alex, Terry Rey, and Sarah J. Mahler. 2009. *Churches and Charity in the Immigrant City: Religion, Immigration, and Civic Engagement in Miami.* New Brunswick, NJ: Rutgers University Press.

Stychin, Carl. 2000. "Consumption, Capitalism, and the Citizen: Sexuality and Equality Rights Discourse in the European Union." In *Social Policy in an Evolving European Union,* edited by Jo Shaw, 259–276. Oxford: Hart Publishing.

Sun, Ken C. 2012. "Fashioning the Reciprocal Norms of Elder Care: A Case of Immigrants in the United States and their Parents in Taiwan." *Journal of Family Issues* 33(9): 1240–1271.

Sung, Kyu-Talk, and MeeHye Kim. 2002. "The Effects of the U.S. Public Welfare System upon Elderly Korean Immigrants' Independent Living Arrangements." *Journal of Poverty* 6(4):83–94.

Taylor, Robert Joseph, Linda M. Chatters, and Jeff Levin. 2004. "Impact of Religion on Mental Health and Well-being." In *Religion in the Lives of African Americans: Social,*

Psychological, and Health Perspectives, edited by Taylor, Chatters, and Levin, 207–226. New Delhi, India: Sage.

Taylor, Robert Joseph, Linda M. Chatters, Jacqueline S. Mattis, and Sean Joe. 2010. "Religious Involvement among Caribbean Blacks in the United States." *Review of Religious Research* 52(2): 125–145.

Templeton, Jacqueline. 2003. *From the Mountains to the Bush: Italian Migrants Write Home from Australia, 1860–1962*. Nedlands, Australia: University of Western Australia Publishing.

Thobani, Sunera. 2007. *Exalted Subjects: Studies in the Making of Race and Nation in Canada*. Toronto: University of Toronto Press.

Thomas, William Isaac, and Florian Znaniecki. [1918] 1996. *The Polish Peasant in Europe and America: Monograph of an Immigrant Group*. Vol. 2. Chicago: University of Chicago Press.

Thompson, Stephanie Lindsay. 1980. *Australia through Italian Eyes: A Study of Settlers Returning from Australia to Italy*. Melbourne: Oxford University Press.

Townson, Monica. 2000. *A Report Card on Women and Poverty*. Ottawa: Canadian Centre Policy Alternatives.

———. 2005. "Poverty Issues for Canadian Women: Background Paper." Status of Women Canada. Available at http://dsp-psd.pwgsc.gc.ca/Collection/SW21-143-2005E.pdf, accessed May 22, 2015.

Treas, Judith. 2008. "Transnational Older Adults and Their Families." *Family Relations* 57: 468–478.

Treas, Judith, and Shampa Mazumdar. 2004. "Kin Keeping and Caregiving: Contributions of Older People in Immigrant Families." *Journal of Comparative Family Studies* 35: 105–122.

Turpel, Mary Ellen. 1993. "Patriarchy and Paternalism: The Legacy of the Canadian State for First Nations Women." *Canadian Journal of Women and the Law* 6(1): 174–192.

Twum-Baah, K. A. 2005. "Volume and Characteristics of International Ghanaian Migration." In *At Home in the World? International Migration and Development in Contemporary Ghana and West Africa*, edited by Takyiwaa Manuh, 55–77. Accra: Sub-Saharan Publishers.

Twum Baah, K. A., J. S. Nabila, and A. F. Aryee, eds. 1995. *Migration Research Study in Ghana*. Accra: Ghana Statistical Service.

U.N. Data. 2012. "Composition of Macro Geographical (Continental) Regions, Geographical Sub-regions, and Selected Economic and Other Groupings." Available at http://millenniumindicators.un.org/unsd/methods/m49/m49regin.htm accessed May 13, 2014.

Urry, John. 2003. "Social Networks, Travel, and Talk." *The British Journal of Sociology* 54(2): 155–175.

van der Geest, Sjaak. 1997. "Money and Respect: The Changing Value of Old Age in Rural Ghana." *Africa* 67(4): 534–559.

———. 2002. "Respect and Reciprocity: Care of Elderly People in Ghana." *Journal of Cross-Cultural Gerontology* 17: 3–31.

van der Geest, Sjaak, Anke Mul, and Hans Vermeulen. 2004. "Linkages between Migration and the Care of Frail Older People: Observations from Greece, Ghana, and the Netherlands." *Aging and Society* 24(3): 431–450.

van Dijk, Rijk. 2002. "Religion, Reciprocity, and Restructuring Family Responsibility in the Ghanaian Pentecostal Diaspora." In *The Transnational Family*, edited by Deborah Bryceson and Ulla Vuorela, 173–196. New York: Berg.

van Nes, Fenna, Tineke Abma, Hans Jonsson, and Dorly Deeg. 2010. "Language Differences in Qualitative Research: Is Meaning Lost in Translation?" *European Journal of Ageing* 7: 313–316.

Varma, Pavan K. 1998. *The Great Indian Middle Class.* Delhi: Penguin.

Vera-Sanso, Penny. 1999. "Dominant Daughters-in-Law and Submissive Mothers-in-Law? Co-operation and Conflict in South India." *Journal of the Royal Anthropological Institute* 5(4): 577–593.

Verjee, Begum. 2012. "Critical Race Feminism: A Transformative Vision for Service-Learning Engagement." *Journal of Community Engagement and Scholarship* 5(1): 57–69.

Vertovec, Steven. 2009. *Transnationalism.* New York: Routledge.

Villalpando, Octavio, and Dolores Delgado Bernal. 2002. "A Critical Race Theory Analysis of Barriers That impede the Success of Faculty of Color." In *The Racial Crisis in American Higher Education: Continuing Challenges for the Twenty-first Century*, edited by William A. Smith, Philip G. Altbach, and Kofi Lomotey, 243–270. Albany: State University of New York Press.

Waldinger, Roger, and Michael I. Lichter. 2003. *How the Other Half Works: Immigration and the Social Organization of Labor.* Berkeley: University of California Press.

Wang, Leslie. 2010. "Importing Western Childhoods into a Chinese State-Run Orphanage." *Qualitative Sociology* 33: 137–159.

Warin, Megan, and Simone Dennis. 2008. "Telling Silences: Unspeakable Trauma and the Unremarkable Practices of Everyday Life." *Sociological Review* 56: 100–116.

Weeks, Kathi. 2011. *The Problem with Work: Feminism, Marxism, Antiwork Politics, and Postwork Imaginaries.* Durham, NC: Duke University Press.

Weerasinghe, Swarna, and Matthew Numer. 2011. "A Life-Course Exploration of the Social, Emotional, and Physical Health Behaviours of Widowed South Asian Immigrant Women in Canada: Implications for Health and Social Programme Planning." *International Journal of Migration, Health, and Social Care* 6(4): 42–56.

West, Candace, and Don H. Zimmerman. 1987. Doing Gender. *Gender and Society* 1(2):125–151.

Williams, David, and Ruth Williams-Morris. 2002. "Racism and Mental Health: The African American Experience." *Ethnicity and Health* 5(3/4): 243–268.

Williams, Fiona. 2011. Markets and migrants in the care economy. *Soundings* 47(8): 22–3.

Williams, Patricia J. 1991. *The Alchemy of Race and Rights.* Cambridge, MA: Harvard University Press.

Wilson-Ford, Vanessa. 1990. "Poverty among Black Elderly Women." *Journal of Women and Aging* 2(4): 5–20.

Wing, Adrien Katherine. 1997. "Introduction." In *Critical Race Feminism: A Reader*, edited by Adrien K. Wing, 1–6. 1st ed. New York: New York University Press.

———. 2003. "Introduction." In *Critical Race Feminism: A Reader*, edited by Adrien K. Wing, 1–19. 2nd ed. New York: New York University Press.

World Bank. 2011. *Migration and Remittances Factbook 2011.* 2nd ed. Washington, DC: World Bank.

Wright, Bernadette. 2005. "Direct Care Workers in Long-Term Care." Washington, DC: AARP Public Policy Institute.

Wu, Yuping, Xiaoyu Han, and Qin Gao. 2005. *Jiating Jiyang: Dongji yu Jixiao* [Family fostering: motivation and effect]. Beijing: Social Sciences Academic Press.

Wu, Zheng, and Randy Hart. 2002. "Social and Health Factors Associated with Support among Elderly Immigrants in Canada." *Research on Aging* 24(4): 391–412.

Xiao, Yuchun, and Fang Lee Cooke. 2012. "Work-Life Balance in China? Social Policy, Employer Strategy, and Individual Coping Mechanisms." *Asia Pacific Journal of Human Resources* 50(1): 6–22.

Yan, Yunxiang. 2003. *Private Life under Socialism.* Stanford, CA: Stanford University Press.

————. 2010. "Introduction: Conflicting Images of the Individual and Contested Process of Individualization." In *China: The Rise of the Modern Chinese Society*, edited by Mette Halskov Hansen, and Rene Svarverud, 1–38. Copenhagen: NIAS Press.

————. 2011a. "The Individualization of the Family in Rural China." *Boundary* 38(1): 203–229.

————. 2011b. "The Changing Moral Landscape." In *Deep China*, edited by Arthur Kleinman et al., 36–77. Berkeley: University of California Press.

Yarris, Kristin Elizabeth. 2014a. "'Pensando Mucho' ('Thinking Too Much'): Embodied Distress among Grandmothers in Nicaraguan Transnational Families." *Culture, Medicine, and Psychiatry* 38: 473–498.

————. 2014b. "'Quiero ir y no quiero ir': (I want to go and I don't want to go): Nicaraguan Children's Ambivalent Experiences of Transnational Family Life." *Journal of Latin American and Caribbean Anthropology* 19(2): 284–309.

Yeates, Nicola. 2005. "A Global Political Economy of Care." *Social Policy & Society* 4(2):227–234.

————. 2009. *Globalizing Care Economies and Migrant Workers: Explorations in Global Care Chains.* New York: Palgrave Macmillan.

Zelizer, Viviana A. 2005. *The Purchase of Intimacy.* Princeton, NJ: Princeton University Press.

Zentgraf, Kristine M., and Norma Stoltz Chinchilla. 2012. "Transnational Family Separation: A Framework for Analysis." *Journal of Ethnic and Migration Studies* 38(2): 345–366.

Zhan, Heying Jenny, and Rhonda J. V. Montgomery. 2003. "Gender and Elder Care in China: The Influence of Filial Piety and Structural Constraints." *Gender and Society* 17(2): 209–229.

Zhang, Hong. 2004. "'Living Alone' and the Rural Elderly: Strategy and Agency in Post-Mao Rural China." In *Filial Piety*, edited by Charlotte Ikels, 63–87. Stanford, CA: Stanford University Press.

————. 2005. "Bracing for an Uncertain Future: A Case Study of New Coping Strategies of Rural Parents under China's Birth Control Policy." *China Journal* 54: 53–76.

Zhou, Yanqiu Rachel. 2012. "Space, Time, and Self: Rethinking Aging in the Contexts of Immigration and Transnationalism." *Journal of Aging Studies* 26(3): 232–242.

————. 2013. "Toward Transnational Care Interdependence: Rethinking the Relationships between Care, Immigration, and Social Policy." *Global Social Policy* 13(3): 280–298.

ABOUT THE CONTRIBUTORS

LORETTA BALDASSAR is discipline chair of Anthropology and Sociology at the University of Western Australia and adjunct principal research fellow, School of Political and Social Inquiry, Monash University. She has published extensively on transnational migrants, families, and caregiving, including *Transnational Families, Migration and the Circulation of Care: Understanding Mobility and Absence in Family Life* (with Laura Merla, 2014) and *Families Caring across Borders* (with Cora Baldock and Raelene Wilding, 2007), as well as many journal articles and book chapters on this subject.

CATI COE is a professor of anthropology at Rutgers University. She is currently working on changes in elder care, including the commercialization of care, in Ghana, as well as on Ghanaians' experiences in elder care work in the United States. She is the author of *The Scattered Family: African Migrants, Parenting and Global Inequality* (2013) and coeditor of *Everyday Ruptures: Children, Youth, and Migration in Global Perspective* (2011) and *The Anthropology of Sibling Relationships: Shared Parentage, Experience and Exchange* (2013).

NEDA DENEVA is a fellow at the International Research Center on Work and the Lifecourse in Global History, Humboldt Universität, Berlin. She holds a PhD in sociology and social anthropology from Central European University. She has worked on Roma and Bulgarian Muslims, exploring the reconfigurations of citizenship by migrants' everyday claims and struggles within the European Union. Her research interests include transnational migration, labor transformations and new work regimes, citizenship and relations with the state. She has publications in the journals *Social Politics, Migrations Societe*, and *Bulgarian Folklore*.

PARIN DOSSA is a professor of anthropology and associate member in the Department of Gender, Sexuality, and Women's Studies at Simon Fraser University. Her ethnographic work has focused on Muslim women in Canada, Lamu

(Kenya), Afghanistan, and more recently, India. Her research interests include displacement, inequality and injustice, structural violence, disability, story-telling, memory work, and diaspora. She is the author of *Politics and Poetics of Migration: Narratives of Iranian Women from the Diaspora* (2004); *Racialized Bodies, Disabling Worlds: Storied Lives of Immigrant Muslim Women* (2009); and *Afghanistan Remembers: Narrations of Violence and Culinary Practices* (2014).

MUSHIRA MOHSIN KHAN is a PhD student in the Department of Sociology and a student affiliate with the Centre on Aging at the University of Victoria. Her research primarily focuses on transnational ties and intergenerational relationships within mid- to later-life diasporic South Asian families, aging, health, and social care. Her work has recently been published in an edited volume on health care equity for ethnic minority older adults (2015), the *Population Change and Lifecourse Strategic Knowledge Cluster Discussion Paper Series*, and the *International Journal of Migration, Health, and Social Care*. She is also the recipient of the Social Sciences and Humanities Research Canada (SSHRC) Joseph-Armand Bombadier Canadian Doctoral Scholarship (2015–2018).

KAREN KOBAYASHI is an associate professor of sociology and research affiliate with the Centre on Aging at the University of Victoria. Her scholarly interests lie broadly in the areas of family and intergenerational relationships, ethnicity and immigration, dementia and personhood, and health and social care. She is currently coediting a forthcoming book on Canadian families in the new millennium (2016) and has recently published work in the *Handbook of Families in Asia, Canadian Families Today: New Perspectives, Multiple Discrimination from an Age Perspective, International Journal of Migration, Health, and Social Care*, the *Journal of Family Issues*, and *Ageing and Society*.

DELORES V. MULLINGS is an associate professor at Memorial University in the School of Social Work. Her scholarly interests include mothering, service learning, teaching and learning, international distance collaborative teaching, health and social needs of older Black and racialized adults, Black queer older adults, critical race theory, anti-Black racism, newcomers in rural and/or small urban centers and racism in Canadian social policy. Recent publications include: "Community Service Learning: A Teaching Tool to help Students Acknowledge Their Own Racism" (2013), "How Black Mothers 'Successfully' Raise Children in the 'Hostile' Canadian Climate" (2013), and "The Racial Institutionalization of Whiteness in Contemporary Canadian Public Policy" (2015).

ERIN L. RAFFETY is a lecturer in the Writing Program at Princeton University whose dissertation in anthropology, "Fostering Family: Kinning Disabled Children in Contemporary China," challenges scholarly claims that insist that the Chinese family is in decline, by detailing creative family-making processes by individuals living on the margins of society. In addition to Chinese studies, Raffety is an expert in the anthropology of childhood, family, gender, and disability, and has recently published an article in the interdisciplinary journal, *Childhood*, which critiques existing participatory methods of doing research with children and advances her own method based on minimizing social distance between researchers and children.

KRISTIN ELIZABETH YARRIS is an assistant professor of International Studies and affiliated faculty in the Department of Anthropology at the University of Oregon. Her research interests include transnational migration and its impacts for care and caregiving, and health and well-being in families, communities, states, and nongovernmental organizations, particularly in Central America and Mexico. She is currently completing a book titled *Solidarity and Care: Grandmothers and Nicaraguan Transnational Families.* Her work has appeared in *Culture, Medicine, and Psychiatry*, the *Journal of Latin American and Caribbean Anthropology*, and *International Migration*, among other venues.

YANQIU RACHEL ZHOU is an associate professor at the Institute on Globalization and the Human Condition and the School of Social Work, McMaster University. Her major research interests include immigration, transnationalism, global health, social policy, and temporalities. She has widely published in edited books and in various peer-reviewed journals, including *Journal of Aging Studies; Health, Time & Society; Globalization; Social Science & Medicine; International Journal of Feminist Approaches to Bioethics; Culture, Health & Sexuality*; and *Global Social Policy.*

INDEX

Printed in the United States
By Bookmasters